ENOUGH OF THE FEAR:

An Insider's Guide to Understanding, Managing, and Living Well with Multiple Sclerosis

Katy Wright, PA-C, Mandy Winkler, RN, and Darin T. Okuda, MD

CONTENTS

Enough of the Fear

1

PREFACE

This book, along with the other digital resources referenced, is intended to provide education only and should not be used as a substitute for professional medical advice. The content contained within may serve as great discussion topics for future medical visits.

Please remember to seek the guidance from your physician and healthcare team before implementing any information that you may have read. The content is also not intended to diagnose, treat, or alter the timing of the delivery of care for your condition in any way.

I focused my career on the study of multiple sclerosis (MS) as I felt it was the only subspecialty in neurology that offered healthcare providers the opportunity to become pioneers, regardless of their time of entry in the field. I still believe this to be true today. During the early days of my journey nearly 17 years ago, the exact cause responsible for the onset of MS was unknown and it still remains a mystery currently. Although tremendous advances have been made over the past fifteen years with an equal number of FDA approved treatments now available to patients aimed at preventing disease advancement, key revisions to our diagnostic criteria made with improvements in diagnostic imaging, changes to the description of the clinical course of MS, and even the identification of new MS subtypes, education continues to serve as a key tenet when navigating this enigmatic condition. Throughout my interaction with a wealth of patients with varying backgrounds and clinical experiences, I am more clear on the type of information that patients desire and truly need.

The idea for this project was conceived after caring for thousands of patients, from those who were newly diagnosed to others with a longstanding history for MS. Although, online MS data are profound with the availability of social media groups and the existence of other online platforms coupled with available resources in app, electronic print, and hard copy form, I felt that the available data were lacking in many practical aspects and, in most cases, they reminded me more of sterile encyclopedia books than immediately intuitive sources of information. More importantly, the content provided seemed to lack the expertise of other members of the healthcare team that are pivotal in the daily care of MS patients – advanced practice providers (i.e. physician assistants and nurse practitioners) and, most importantly, nurses who are corresponding at a higher frequency with our patients than any other member of the healthcare team.

Information that you would not typically expect to find in a conventional MS resource is also provided. Each key section also contains summarized information outlined as 'Helpful Hints', allowing readers to access key points easily.

The intended audience includes those who are new to the diagnosis of MS along with established patients, their family members, healthcare providers, and for those wanting to learn more about this unique condition. In this seminal version of our contemporary resource, the most relevant and meaningful information is provided to readers with information delivered in a way that is concise, efficient, and practical. Although the printed version of our eBook does not allow for immediate access to our online resources, descriptions to additional resources are provided. An earlier iteration of this work involved compiling a resource that was specific to different time points of an individual's experience with MS, from diagnosis to the mid- and later- stages of the condition. However, given how this condition behaves in a way that can be so unpredictable, we managed to design something that is both timeless and universal. The nature of the platform by which this is being delivered will also allow for our team to quickly incorporate new updates occurring within the field of MS.

The future of MS is exceptionally promising and, in my opinion, some of the greatest contributions to science spanning other disciplines will result from work within our field. Treatments extending beyond those aimed at preventing relapses and disability will soon be available, specifically those focused on central nervous system repair. The hope is that the management of MS will mirror other chronic diseases in our field (i.e. hypertension and Type II diabetes mellitus, etc.) that are effectively addressed with interventions beyond prescribed therapies.

Katy, Mandy, and I would like to extend our gratitude to Julie Cox and Jose R. Santoyo for the art work showcased throughout this resource. We would also like to recognize Madison R. Hansen and Braeden D. Newton, two of my former research assistants who now represent the future of medicine, for their invaluable contribution within many chapters.

We are also so very grateful to all of our patients and their family members, colleagues, and our families for providing inspiration for us to complete this work.

D.T.O.

How to Use This Book

This book is designed to provide the most practical information pertaining to multiple sclerosis; it is intended to both educate and demystify.

We will walk you through what we believe is most pertinent to understanding, managing, and living well with MS. Our goal is to synthesize an abundance of information into a single source that is easy to navigate and understand. We hope that this book answers all of your questions - even the ones you haven't thought of yet!

Katy

INTRODUCTION

Multiple sclerosis (MS) is an immune-mediated disorder, similar to rheumatoid arthritis or lupus, where the body's immune system misbehaves and mistakenly attacks healthy cells. In the case of MS, immune cells destroy the protective covering of nerve cells called myelin. Historically, MS has been known principally as a demyelinating disorder, but the damage incurred actually extends beyond the myelin sheath and may involve the nerve fibers themselves and other cell types within the brain! You may hear your provider refer to the disease formally as an inflammatory disorder of the central nervous system (CNS), a system that is comprised of the brain and spinal cord. The brain, optic nerve, and spinal cord are targets in MS. An individual's immune system incorrectly recognizes healthy nerve tissue as foreign leading to inflammation, demyelination, and nerve damage. Injury to myelin impairs the ability for a nerve to communicate effectively. Thus, information traveling from the brain to the body often gets interrupted or delayed. This breakdown in communication can lead to a variety of clinical symptoms that vary from patient to patient.[1,2] This is why everyone's MS is distinctly unique!

What causes MS and who gets it?

There is not a single identifiable cause of MS. As previously mentioned, it is an immune-mediated condition, and certain individuals are genetically predisposed to autoimmune disorders. We find that autoimmune disorders tend to 'cluster' in families. Do any of your relatives have RA, lupus, Crohn's disease, or ulcerative colitis? There are a variety of environmental exposures that can trigger disease activity in those individuals who are susceptible. Exposures that have been of interest include vitamin D deficiency, Epstein-Barr virus infection, diet, vaccinations, air pollutants, and chemical exposures.[3-5]

This condition can occur in any ethnic group but is most common in Caucasians, and among Caucasians, those of northern European decent are at highest risk. However, the prevalence of MS is increasing in many areas across the globe. The Multiple Sclerosis Foundation estimates that approximately 400,000 individuals in the United States are affected by MS, and over 2.5 million people are affected worldwide.[6,7] Most patients are diagnosed as young adults, but the disease can occur in children and later in life. MS is more than twice as likely to occur in women compared to men.[1, 6-8]

Am I going to pass MS down to my children?

Although genetic factors play a role in who develops MS, the disease is not directly passed down from parents to children. There is a slightly higher risk of developing MS for first degree relatives (children, siblings) compared to the general population.[2, 8, 9] The unaffected identical twin who has a sibling with MS has the highest life-time risk followed by children who have both parents with the disease.

Possible Signs of MS

Presenting symptoms of MS are typically unfamiliar and troublesome for the patient and their family members. There is a wide range of non-specific symptoms depending on the location of the inflammation within the nervous system. Some signs may include:

- Numbness or tingling
- Painful vision loss
- Change in color vision
- Double vision or blurry vision
- New onset weakness
- Changes in walking or balance difficulties
- Dizziness

Diagnosing MS

There is no single test available to detect MS. The diagnosis is made through a thorough clinical history, neurological exam, magnetic resonance imaging (MRI) studies, cerebrospinal fluid studies, and blood tests.[2] Individuals must meet formal diagnostic criteria known as the McDonald criteria, fulfilling the requirements for prior clinical experiences and associated findings on MRI studies of the brain and spinal cord.[10] Some diagnostic tests may include:

- ° MRI studies of the brain, cervical spine, and thoracic spine
- ° Optical Coherence Tomography (OCT)
- ° Blood work
- ° Lumbar Puncture
- ° Visual Evoked Potentials

Ruling Out Other Conditions

There are several disorders that can produce neurological symptoms and imaging findings that are similar to those found in MS. Potential mimics include: metabolic disorders, vascular disorders, infections, inflammatory disorders, nutritional deficiencies, and psychiatric illness. For the purposes of this book, we will presume that these conditions have already been excluded.

Helpful Hints:

- ❖ While some physicians may order a lumbar puncture, this test is not required for the diagnosis of MS. The presence of unique oligoclonal bands within the fluid that surrounds your brain and spinal cord (in comparison to bands from your blood sample) and elevated levels of IgG antibodies are indicative of MS, however, many patients with MS may never have these findings.

- ❖ Abnormalities observed on Visual Evoked Potential (VEP) studies are non-specific for MS but can provide supportive data. This test identifies impaired communication along the optic nerve pathways. It is not uncommon for damage to occur along this pathway before patients ever develop visual symptoms.

- ❖ Optical coherence tomography, a non-invasive study of the eyes that aims to assess the integrity of your retinal nerve fiber layer may reveal anatomical changes supportive of the diagnosis of MS.

- ❖ Blood work is typically performed to evaluate for the presence of other conditions (i.e. vitamin and mineral deficiencies, infections, metabolic abnormalities, etc.) that may explain your health challenges. Always keep in mind that multiple autoimmune conditions may be identified.

- ❖ At times patience is needed (which is easier said than done) and information from multiple time points may be required to arrive at an accurate diagnosis

2

SO YOU HAVE MS, NOW WHAT?
Making Your First Appointment

"My primary care physician thinks I have multiple sclerosis. When should I schedule my first visit with a neurologist?"

Early intervention is key in stopping disease progression and preventing long-term disability. So schedule an appointment with a neurologist as soon as possible because there are a variety of EFFECTIVE treatment options available! And, new therapies are being introduced at an increasingly rapid rate.

Appointment availability will be variable depending on the practitioner. It is not uncommon for some physicians to schedule new patient appointments several months in advance while other providers may be able to accommodate appointments right away. Regardless of when you are able to see a neurologist, being prepared for your initial visit is critical. Great resources are available when developing strategies prior to your first visit, allowing you to understand what to expect during your evaluation, and how to determine success afterwards (search Pre-Meet: Multiple Sclerosis in the App Store or Google Play).

Choosing Your Provider

As you embark on this journey, it is important to consider the patient-provider relationship. It is, after all, the heart of medicine. Because MS is a lifelong neurologic disorder, you will be spending a considerable amount of time with your health-care team, and you want to establish a meaningful relationship. There are several factors to consider in order to optimize this connection.

It is well worth your time to take a few minutes to reflect on what kind of patient you are. Do you believe the doctor always knows best? Does he/she have all the right answers and make all of the decisions on your behalf? Is it important for you that your physician use new medical technology? Should they be actively involved in clinical research? Use the newest medical therapies? Or, do you believe you know your body best?

Some patients prefer to take the lead and like to make their own decisions when it comes to their health. Would you prefer your provider to have minimal involvement? Would you work best with someone who allows you to make as many choices as medically reasonable? Or, do you sit somewhere in the middle where you value your physician's expertise and guidance, but you want to be included in the decision-making process? These are important questions to ask yourself before establishing care with a physician.

You must also consider whether you prefer a single physician practice versus a combination practice that utilizes a healthcare team. The main benefit of a single physician practice is that you see the same provider every visit. You are able to develop a strong bond and working relationship with that individual. The down side to this approach is that if the physician is unavailable, you may be unable to be evaluated in clinic. On the other hand, clinics that use an integrative approach utilize physicians, advanced practice providers (physician assistants and nurse practitioners), dieticians, physical therapists, and other health care providers, which can allow for extra time and attention during office visits. This approach is typically more conducive for comprehensive care. However, based on the evolution of healthcare, it is likely that you will not see your physician at every appointment.

You may end up consulting with several physicians before you find someone who meets your specific needs. You should feel comfortable asking questions and providing input during your visit. If you do not feel comfortable and connected with your physician, it is recommended that you find another provider that you are more compatible with. Your well-being is most important, and do your best to be your own advocate.

"My Internist has referred me to a general neurologist. Do I need to see a MS specialist?"

A general neurologist is a physician who specializes in neurology. They are trained to treat a broad range of neurologic conditions. Specialists involved in the care of MS patients are board certified neurologists who may or may not have completed a fellowship specific to neuroimmunological disorders. They are considered the experts in the field and are abreast with the latest information including data from recent research studies, the latest in symptom management as well as emerging therapies. If you feel as if your general neurologist is unable to adequately care for you, request a referral to a MS specialist. A one-time consultation may be performed (with or without the knowledge of your existing doctor) and you may then determine if a transfer of care of necessary. Alternatively, many patients are evaluated by specialists annually for new insights into their disorder and continue to have their care provided by their general neurologist.

Helpful Hints:

❖ Ask your primary care physician for recommendations and/or referrals for a neurologist in your area. The National MS Society has a 'Find a Neurologist' tool that may be helpful as well.

❖ Consider how far you are willing to travel to be seen. Your provider will request that you come in for routine follow-up appointments and diagnostic testing. Alternatively, once-a-year visits with a specialist may also be considered while routinely being cared for by your local health care programs.

❖ Seek recommendations from friends or local support groups.

Preparing for Your First Appointment

With the current state of health care, individuals must take increasing responsibility for their care. Once you have scheduled your first appointment, make sure to collect your records from previous health care providers (i.e. office notes, MRI CDs, lab results, etc). Do not rely on the medical records departments from outside healthcare institutions to compile and distribute your records for you. It is not uncommon for paperwork to get lost in the shuffle, so it is important for you to have a copy of your records as well.

In order for your visit to run smoothly, you must be equipped with questions and with a clear timeline of your clinical events and previous diagnostic workup. A lot of information needs to be covered in a short period of time especially on your first visit. Optimize that time by being organized and prepared. While this is likely highly emotional time for you, try your best to be even-tempered during your appointment. When we are engrossed in our emotions, we are not able to fully listen and process information. For this reason, it is always helpful to bring someone with you to your appointment. A condensed summary of strategies when preparing for your first visit may be found here (search Pre-Meet: Multiple Sclerosis in the App Store or Google Play).

Helpful Hints:

❖ Be punctual. Arriving to your appointment early is essential. This will allow for ample time to complete any necessary paperwork prior to your appointment. Allow approximately 30 minutes to complete these tasks.

❖ Consider traffic patterns and parking/valet availability. There may be additional delays depending on the time of your appointment.

❖ Imaging studies not pertaining to your brain or spinal cord is likely not relevant. Do not bring extraneous imaging studies; these are better addressed by the appropriate specialist.

❖ Excessive information will likely impede the progress of your visit, so try to create a concise timeline including only the most relevant information.

❖ Many facilities do charge a fee to obtain medical records, so please be aware. This can often be bypassed if you have your physician request records be sent to the neurologist directly. Always call to ensure records have been received prior to your appointment. There is nothing more frustrating for you or the provider than an unproductive visit.

❖ This will be a professional, working relationship, so treat it as such. Be respectful of the provider's time and of the other patients who have appointments after you.

❖ Always bring your current medical and prescription insurance cards along with a photo I.D. to each visit.

❖ Be prepared to provide the contact information for your preferred pharmacy at the time of your visit so that any prescription medications may be sent directly to your pharmacy.

❖ Bring a list of all of your current medications including the dose and frequency. Some clinics may ask you to bring your medication(s) to your appointment.

❖ Dress appropriately for your appointments. Consider wearing layers because most medical offices are cold. Furthermore, your provider will likely be doing a neurological assessment at most office visits. This may require taking off your socks and shoes or rolling up your pant legs. Do your best to wear clothes that are conducive to this.

❖ Consider bringing someone with you to your appointment. A lot of information will be covered, and a second set of ears is always helpful.

Making the Most of Your Relationship with Your Providers:

Write questions or concerns down between visits so that you do not forget them.

If you have a grievance with your provider (anything from issues with time spent in the waiting room to not having phone calls returned or medications refilled), it is important to address your complaints sooner rather than later. You do not want unaddressed concerns to fester.
Call the provider's office if you have medically related questions that cannot wait until the next visit.

The presence of specific symptoms may be worrisome and it is recommended that you call your specialist if present for > 24 hours.

New or worsening weakness
Changes in your walking or balance
Changes in vision or eye pain
New numbness or tingling
Difficulty with speech or swallowing
New onset dizziness
Change in bowel or bladder function
Change in memory or thinking speed

Please be aware that certain questions are not possible to address over the phone. Your nurse or provider may request that you come in for a sooner appointment to meet with your provider in person.

It is important to remember that not every physical ailment is related to MS. It is best to initially contact your primary care physician before phoning your neurologist with new or worsening symptoms (refer to the symptom guide above).

Fever, flu, cough or sore throat
Constipation or diarrhea
Rash
Vomiting or upset stomach
Urinary tract infections
Muscle aches

Don't reject medical recommendations from your provider unless you have a specific medical or personal reason to do so. In these instances, make sure you discuss your concerns openly with your provider before disregarding their advice.

Always bring an updated medication list to each of your appointments. It is important that your neurologist know what medications other providers have initiated or adjusted.

Make sure you understand dosing instructions and side effects for new medications prior to leaving your appointment. It is easier to ask for clarification while you are still in the office

3

MAKING SENSE OF YOUR DIAGNOSIS

You have met with your neurologist and received the results from your MRIs and other diagnostic studies, and now you have a confirmed diagnosis of MS. This information has begun to sink in, and now you are left trying to wrap your mind around your new diagnosis. How will your life change in the upcoming weeks? Years? The lives of your family members and loved ones? How will you cope with a chronic disease? Know that it's completely normal to experience a range of emotions following a new diagnosis! Anxiety and disbelief will likely be abundant, but there is hope.

You will be able to manage this disease while continuing to live a fulfilling and productive life! The reality is that MS is just another one of life's circumstances that is out of your control. Even though you are just now receiving the diagnosis of MS, it is likely that you have had the disease for a number of years without ever even knowing it. There's nothing you could have done differently to prevent or anticipate your diagnosis, so don't beat yourself up!

While you did not choose this disease, you do have the power to choose how you respond. Given the scientific advancements related to the care of MS, you do not have to worry excessively or become overwhelmed. Newly diagnosed patients frequently express that they feel as if they have lost all sense of control over their lives, but remember knowledge is power. You now have the opportunity to intervene with effective treatments and change the course of your disease!

It is important to identify your thoughts and become aware of your feelings, after all, this is what determines your actions. Understanding your emotions can help you gain a sense of control. We have identified some of the most common fears experienced by newly diagnosed patients, which are outlined below.

Most Common Fears

Fear of the unknown is by far the biggest apprehension that newly diagnosed patients express to me. However, it is possible to live a rewarding life despite a seemingly uncertain future. MS is an unpredictable disease, and it varies from patient to patient, but over time, patients learn patterns of their own individual disease and symptoms. Be your best champion. Learning these patterns is a process. It takes time to adjust, and living in the unsettled, mysterious space of the unknown is difficult. Nonetheless, it does get better! You may eventually establish a new normal and carry on with your daily routines. Alternatively, you may feel no different than you did prior to your diagnosis and having MS may serve as an excellent catalyst for propelling your general health.

Another recurring source of angst, is the fear of future disability. A large majority of patients associate the diagnosis of MS with a future life sentence to a wheelchair or a walker. This is NOT the case, especially with the availability of a wealth of treatments that have been shown to reduce physical disability over time. While the fear of ambulatory difficulties is a valid concern, our goal with current treatments is to intervene early in the disease course to prevent future physical impairments while preserving your quality of life. Treatment options have improved dramatically over the course of the past twenty years. We now have effective treatment options that can help prevent future disability, which was previously not the case. Having MS does not mean that you will end up in a wheelchair.

Most individuals who are diagnosed with MS, at one time or another, fear that they are going to be a burden to those they love most. Regardless of your age at the time of diagnosis, most adults are used to being independent, contributing members of society. They are not accustomed to relying on others for support whether that be emotional, physical, or social, and thus, they fear being an inconvenience to their loved ones. You may not want to ask friends to watch your kids during doctor's appointments or ask for help during carpool and soccer practice, but the reality is, those who love you are willing to help.

Another common source of anxiety for patients is the cost of the illness. MS is an expensive disease, and as you are accepting the news of your diagnosis, you are likely beginning to receive countless bills in the mail as well. As you listen to your physician discuss medications, MRIs, and lab work, you are likely hearing $$$ and worrying about your financial obligations. Disease modifying therapies are expensive medications not to mention the cost of other prescription medications, diagnostic tests, office visit co-insurance payments, physical therapy, and possible hospital admissions. The financial requirements may seem endless, especially initially. Take a deep breath. It will all be okay. There are financial assistance programs, non-profit organizations, and other resources available for patients, which will be addressed in more detail later in this book. Also, keep in mind that what is most important is what your out-of-pocket cost is, not what it costs your insurance provider!

Finally, a common fear that is frequently encountered among newly diagnosed patients, is the fear of others' opinion of the disease. The public's perception of MS has not progressed at the same rate as science. Having MS is no longer a disability sentence as we just discussed. This is one aspect that you have virtually no control over, so it is not worth expending extensive amounts of emotional energy trying to reconcile others' expectations.

Coping Strategies

Facing your diagnosis head on and working with your physician to develop a plan of action is the best way to face your diagnosis. Focus on the aspects of your health that you can control. While you may not be able to alter your diagnosis, you can choose to start on a disease modifying therapy and start making healthy life style modifications. Denial and avoidance place you at greater risk for further emotional distress.

Consider reducing unnecessary obligations and commitments. Now is not the time to head up volunteer organizations or the PTA. Focus on creating a support network for yourself so that you have friends to call upon when needed. Surround yourself with positive and supportive people who will love you and encourage you along the way. Make yourself a priority!

Not to spoil the ending, but everything is going to be alright. Being courageous does not always involve daring actions. Sometimes asking for help and embracing gracious "nos" is the bravest thing you can do.

Helpful Hints:

- ❖ Do not deny or avoid your diagnosis. If you have uncertainty regarding the accuracy of your diagnosis, seek a second opinion.

- ❖ Work with your provider to develop an action plan and focus on the variables that you can control.

❖ Improving your general health is essential for MS patients.

❖ Start creating a support network and integrate those people into your daily life.

4

WHAT'S HAPPENING BEHIND THE SCENES

As previously mentioned, MS is an immune mediated disorder that may cause progressive neurological disability. The immune system is comprised of a complex network of cells and proteins within the body. White blood cells (WBCs) offer the greatest protection against infection. They work by traveling through the body looking for intruders like viruses and bacteria. T-cells and B-cells are both types of WBCs that help protect the body against infections. The immune system is also involved in cancer prevention by destroying both cancerous and precancerous cells. In MS patients, for reasons that are not entirely understood, these cells become confused and overactive. They mistakenly attack myelin within the CNS, which then leaves the exposed nerve vulnerable to injury.[1, 11] As a consequence, the nerve itself may also be damaged, both immediately during an acute inflammatory episode and after time.

Definitions

T cells and B cells are different types of white blood cells that play an active role in the inflammatory process of MS.

Myelin is the protein sheath wrapped around nerve axons that provides protection, insulation, and improves the conduction of signals along nerves.

Oligodendrocytes are the cells that manufacture and maintain the myelin around axons.

Axons are the portion of a nerve cell that carry the electrical impulses (signals).

There is an acute inflammatory phase in MS in which immune cells (T cells and B cells) are able to enter into the CNS. The reasons related to why these cells get stimulated prior to entering the CNS is unclear, however exposure to viruses, bacteria, fungi, things we inhale from the environment along with what we eat may be significant contributors! Once these immune cells are exposed to the brain and spinal cord, an inflammatory cascade ensues damaging the myelin, oligodendrocytes, and ultimately the nerve axons. Following the inflammatory phase, there is a chronic phase that is characterized by deterioration (atrophy) of the previously damaged nerves. This stage of the disease is typically associated with greater physical disability and functional decline.[11, 12]

INJURY TO MYELIN

Myelin is the initial target of the aberrant immune cells, but oligodendrocytes (myelin producing cells) and nerve axons also incur damage from the inflammatory cascade carried out by these cells. (view section on Injury in MS)

Multiple sclerosis has traditionally been categorized into distinct disease courses. These classifications are based on the temporal profile of relapses and disability progression.[13] However, as we learn more about the disease, we are moving away from these somewhat antiquated classifications because each sub-type seems to be more similar than previously suggested.

RADIOLOGICALLY ISOLATED SYNDROME

Radiologically isolated syndrome is an entity in which features highly suggestive of MS are observed incidentally after a brain MRI study is performed for a reason other than for the evaluation of demyelinating disease.[14] These individuals have not yet experienced clinical attacks related to myelin injury. Brain MRI studies are performed for headache, trauma, evaluation of endocrine disorders, curiosity (i.e. mother or sibling with MS), following the study of healthy control subjects for research, etc. This recognized subtype supports the notion that MS is a "silent thief" of neurological well-being, damaging myelin and nerves even before someone experiences a first clinical attack. As many brain MRI studies may reveal the presence of white matter involvement due to headache, aging, high blood pressure, etc., care must be exercised when concluding that the observed changes are truly related to demyelinating disease.

CLINICALLY ISOLATED SYNDROME

Clinically isolated syndrome subjects are individuals who have experienced a clinical attack highly suggestive for MS but fail to meet full criteria for relapsing remitting MS. These patients have a history of a single attack only and symptoms may include vision loss, weakness involving an arm or leg or both legs, numbness and tingling at the torso or extremities, etc. Not all patients who experience a single event go on to develop clinically definite MS. Based on the most recent diagnostic criteria for MS, if 1 or more lesions are observed on repeat MRI testing or if another clinical attack is experienced, that individual would now fulfill the diagnosis of MS.[15, 16]

RELAPSING REMITTING MS

Relapsing remitting MS (RRMS) is the most common form experienced by patients. Early stages of the disease are characterized by episodes of acute inflammation and neurologic dysfunction. For patients, this can manifest as a variety of neurological symptoms such as numbness, weakness, vision loss, etc. This is followed by varying degrees of symptomatic recovery over the course of weeks to months. Deficits incurred during a relapse may resolve entirely but often times there is some degree of residual injury. With each relapse, persistent symptoms tend to accumulate over time. Without medical intervention, relapses occur at variable intervals each year depending on the patient. These relapses are followed by interludes of disease quiescence commonly known as remissions.[17, 18] Remissions can last anywhere from months to years.

SECONDARY PROGRESSIVE MS

Secondary progressive MS (SPMS) follows the relapsing remitting course of the disease. This phase of the disease does not have periods of distinct remissions; it is characterized by a gradual, progressive decline in function. Neurological difficulties accumulate over time and lead to physical disability.[17, 18] Prior scientific data suggests that within 20 years of diagnosis with RRMS, 30-60% of patients convert to SPMS. With advances made in available treatments, a significantly lower rate is being observed! The frequency and severity of disease, including the number of attacks, degree of recovery, and MRI behavior during the relapsing phase of the disease can strongly influence one's likelihood of conversion.[19, 20]

PRIMARY PROGRESSIVE MS

This primary progressive MS (PPMS) experience varies from the others in that symptom(s) progressively worsen from the very beginning. Patients never experience distinct relapses or periods of symptomatic recovery. These patients steadily accumulate disability throughout the course of their disease and only experience infrequent, temporary improvements or plateaus of their symptoms.[17-19] A common example includes weakness at a single leg. Since symptom onset, there is history of a continued decline in strength. Patients need to experience a decline for at least 1-year (along with meeting imaging criteria) to be diagnosed with PPMS. Before just recently, none of our available therapies were FDA approved to treat progressive disease, but now we have a highly effective therapy to treat these patients. Some patients who were on therapy even noticed improvement in their disability! We will discuss available therapies and treatment strategies in detail in Chapter 4.

The clinical course of MS was redefined in 2013, to more accurately describe patient experiences.[21] Disease activity, defined by clinical relapses and/or MRI activity were incorporated into the some of the descriptions above (i.e. relapsing-remitting disease – not active or active, etc.). For those with progressive accumulation of disability from onset or after an initial relapsing course, the term 'progressive disease' with or without activity and progression was introduced.

"How do I know if I have secondary progressive MS?"

This question is best answered retrospectively. If you have noticed a slow, steady decline in your symptoms without intervals of improvement, you have likely entered into the progressive phase. Keep in mind, however, that poor general health is a common contributor to patients not doing well. This alone may make it appear as if a person is entering this phase of the disease state when in fact other contributors are present! Sadly, we're all not getting younger too! Your MS specialist will be able to provide the proper education and reasons for why you may not be feeling as strong as you did earlier.

"Will I end up in a wheelchair?"

No one can precisely predict the answer to this question, but your healthcare team will fight damn hard to ensure this does not happen. Lesions that occur in the spinal cord are typically associated with more walking difficulties, so patients with a high proportion of spinal cord lesions are more likely to require assistive devices. There are exciting treatments on the horizon that aim to repair myelin. These new therapies provide a new approach towards minimizing this risk. For now, physical exercises, including weight lifting is ideal to enhance the reorganization of networks from your spinal cord to your brain.

INJURY IN MULTIPLE SCLEROSIS

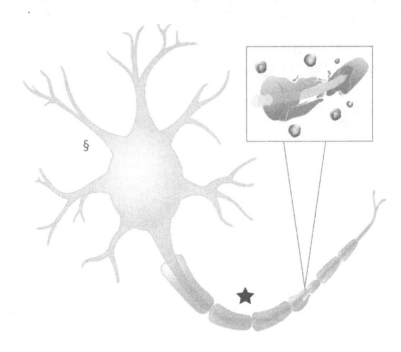

Anatomy of nerve cell body (§), axon (nerve fiber,★), and myelin (pictured in blue). Both B and T cells play a role in the injury of the fatty, insulating layer surrounding the axon (inset). The exact cause amongst all MS patients that results in excitation of the immune system resulting in autoimmune injury is unknown. Injury to myelin and axons may result in the disruption of nerve impulses.

5

UNDERSTANDING MEDICATIONS THAT CAN ALTER YOUR DISEASE

Prior to 1993, there were no available therapies for the treatment of MS. Patients' day-to-day symptoms were managed as best they could, but lacking were medications that had the ability to alter the course of the disease process, prevent MRI changes, relapses, and disability. Since the early 1990s, several therapies have been introduced that aim to prevent relapses and disease progression. These will be referred to as disease modifying therapies (DMTs).[22] These treatments may be injected both into the muscle or fat and are available in pill form or by infusion. It is important to highlight that the frequency by which these treatments are administered vary greatly along with how they are tolerated by patients.

This chapter will focus on the immunosuppressive and immunomodulatory treatments that target certain aspects of the immune system, ultimately, reducing the frequency and severity of relapses as well as future neurological impairments. What's the difference between these two types of treatments? Immunosuppressive agents cause cell death whereas immunomodulatory treatments impact chemokines, fancy chemical mediators that our bodies generate to alter the behavior of immune cells.

It is important to understand that permanent damage can occur early in the disease course. Even when you are asymptomatic and feeling well, irrevocable injury could be occurring to your brain and spinal cord behind the scenes. This is why MS really is a 'silent thief', affecting the integrity of cells and nerves well before the occurrence of a first symptom. Effective therapy is essential early in the disease course to disrupt the inflammatory cascade because, if left unaddressed, it may ultimately end in irreversible injury and subsequent disability.

There are a variety of factors to consider when you discuss starting one of the available approved DMTs with your provider. Thanks to scientific advances, there are an assortment of options and the conversation can be overwhelming. No medication is perfect, but you should be able to agree upon a treatment that you are comfortable with and that fits into your current lifestyle. The best medication on paper, meaning one with the strongest effect on suppressing disease, may not be ideal for you.

When considering a new therapy, efficacy of the medication should be one of the primary considerations. The more efficacious the medication, the greater your chances are for reducing relapses and halting progression early in the disease course, which correlates to more favorable long-term outcomes. However, a proper understanding of risk versus benefit of all treatments should be considered. Also, our need for more 'aggressive' treatments is more likely to occur earlier in the disease course and during our younger years rather than later in life. For the purposes of this book, we will not focus much on medication efficacy as that is a conversation better had with your medical provider in person.

Each medication has its own safety and side effect profile. Ideally, the benefits of the medication that you and your physician select should outweigh the risks, and your specialist may determine this based on the experiences you have had along with the findings on your MRI studies. You must also consider the convenience of the medication and ease of administration. Like any medicine, your disease modifying therapy will only be beneficial if taken as prescribed. That being said, set yourself up for success. Do not consider a therapy that you cannot be compliant with in the long run. Keep in mind that the best therapy is one that you would be willing to take long-term.

Finally, it is crucial to have realistic expectations when starting your new therapy. DMTs are preventative treatments like medications that lower blood pressure or cholesterol. Their goal is to prevent future disease activity. Typically, these medications do not repair damage or restore lost function; however, some of the newer agents may play a role in myelin repair. Additionally, they do not address symptomatic complaints like numbness, tingling, muscle spasms, or muscle weakness. It is important to highlight that some of the newer treatments offered by infusion have been shown to improve disability measures after treatment start. This means that a proportion of patients actually improve neurologically with strength, sensation, vision, cognition, etc. after the start of the treatment. Knowing these things prior to starting your new treatment, will help prevent frustration and disappointment. Ideally, you should not experience any negative side effects once you start on your DMT.

Helpful Hints:

❖ The primary goal of MS therapy is to prevent premature disability and to preserve quality of life outcomes. This goal is, in part, achieved through the prevention of new clinical attacks and new MRI lesions.

❖ DMTs are not primarily designed to make you feel better. They do not typically address symptomatic complaints like pain, weakness, or fatigue. There are other therapies designed to target those concerns. However, keep in mind that some of the available treatments are associated with improvements in neurological function.

❖ Our current therapies do not substantially reverse or heal damage that has incurred from previous relapses. This highlights the importance of relapse prevention!

❖ It is not uncommon for patients to have breakthrough disease on one or more therapies. Do not be discouraged if this is the case for you too. It may take several DMT changes before finding the one you respond to best.

❖ Once you start on therapy, you will need to have routine lab work, clinical visits, and surveillance MRIs to gauge how well you are responding to treatment.

AVAILABLE THERAPIES

There are currently fifteen FDA approved disease modifying therapies available for the treatment of relapsing remitting multiple sclerosis, and there are even more currently in development. We will provide a brief overview of the existing therapies.

INJECTABLE THERAPIES

These were the first medications introduced in the early 1990s and have historically been referred to as the ABC drugs. These are subcutaneous and intramuscular injections that are administered at varying frequencies depending on the medication. They all come available with auto injectors and in pre-filled syringes to make taking the medication as stress-free as possible.

INTERFERONS

Interferons are small molecules called cytokines that are naturally produced by our own immune system in response to a variety of stressor such as viral infections. They have inherent immuno-modulatory properties that help temper immune responses. This medication works by influencing the transportation of immune cells into the central nervous system and altering some of the proteins produced by certain white blood cells (T cells and B cells). Side effects are somewhat dependent on the dosing and frequency of the medication. Flu-like symptoms such as fever, chills, and body aches are the most common side effects of the interferons. These typically last for 24-48 hours following the injections. Patients may also experience injection site reactions (pain, redness, tenderness, swelling). Less common side effects include mood changes, thyroid dysfunction, elevated liver enzymes, and a decline in white blood cell counts. Thus, routine lab work is recommended to follow these values.[23-31]

	FDA Approval	Dose/Route	Frequency
Betaseron	1993	250mcg subcutaneous	every other day
Avonex	1996	30mcg intramuscular	once a week
Rebif	2002	44mcg subcutaneous	three times weekly
Extavia	2009	250mcg subcutaneous	every other day
Plegridy	2014	125mcg subcutaneous	every other week

Helpful Hints:

❖ Flu like side effects are very common. These typically improve over time. Pre-treating with acetaminophen and ibuprofen prior to your injections will help minimize these symptoms. Your provider can also give you a prescription anti-inflammatory if over the counter medications are not helpful.

❖ Drinking extra water and eating foods high in potassium the day of your injections can also help to minimize side effects.

❖ If you have side effects, it may be helpful to take your injections at bedtime so that you are asleep when symptoms are at their peak.

❖ These medications are started at a smaller dose and are incrementally increased to help minimize side effects.

❖ Patients can develop antibodies to interferon, which negate the immunomodulatory effects of the medications. Your physician should periodically check for neutralizing antibodies.

GLATIRAMER ACETATE (COPAXONE)

Glatiramer acetate (Copaxone, Glatopa, glatiramer acetate) is a synthetic copolymer that mimics myelin basic protein (part of the myelin sheath). It is thought to inhibit T cells from damaging myelin of the central nervous system although the exact mechanism of action is still not fully understood. It has a favorable safety and side effect profile with injection site reactions being the most common side effect. However, there is a rare systemic reaction characterized by palpitations, chest pain, and shortness of breath. This is a spontaneous reaction that is not harmful and self resolves within 30-45 minutes although it can be rather alarming to patients and their loved ones. Routine lab work is not required for this medication but is ultimately left to the discretion of your provider.[32-34]

	FDA Approval	Dose/Route	Frequency
Copaxone	1996	20mg subcutaneous	daily
Copaxone	2014	40mg subcutaneous	thrice weekly
Glatopa	2015	20mg subcutaneous	daily
glatiramer acetate	2017	20mg subcutaneous	daily
glatiramer acetate	2017	40mg subcutaneous	thrice weekly

Helpful Hints:

❖ Glatiramer acetate is one of the safest MS medications available. So, if safety is important to you, it may be a good fit for you initially.

❖ Given the complex nature of the synthetic proteins that comprise the name brand medication, it is thought that the generic formulation of the medication may not be as effective.

❖ To improve tolerability, allow the medication to come to room temperature before injecting. Topical hydrocortisone and Benadryl cream may also help improve injection site reactions.

❖ If you are having difficulty with your injections, repeating injections training with a nurse may be of value to help improve your technique

❖ If your injections are overly painful, ask your provider if you are a candidate for lidocaine or another numbing cream to use prior to injections.

❖ Be mindful that more generic offerings of glatiramer acetate are available with lower annual retail costs than Copaxone. As a result, some insurance providers may require patients to switch to these non-branded formulations.

DACLIZUMAB (ZINBRYTA)

Daclizumab was one of the newly introduced MS medications that was approved for use in the U.S. in 2016. The medication targeted specific T cells (CD 25 cells), impairing their inflammatory function. It was self-administered by subcutaneous injection once a month. The most common side effects from the clinical trials were upper respiratory infections, flu, rash (dry, itchy skin), and elevated liver enzymes on routine lab work. Due to the immunosuppressive nature of the medication, it had the potential of causing reactivation of latent infections such as tuberculosis or hepatitis. In early 2018, drug manufacturers, Biogen and AbbVie, voluntarily removed this medication from the market due to concerns over safety. Liver injury and immune mediated conditions (i.e. encephalitis and meningoencephalitis) were of primary concern.

ORAL THERAPIES

FINGOLIMOD (GILENYA)

Fingolimod (Gilenya) was the first oral medication, introduced in 2010. It is a once daily pill that works by isolating lymphocytes (a type of white blood cell) in the lymph nodes. It's believed that the sequestering of these cells prevents them from entering the central nervous system and subsequently causing an inflammatory response. This will cause a reduction in total white blood cell count and absolute lymphocyte counts, which is monitored with routine blood tests.

Gilenya is a very well tolerated medication and has very few side effects on a day to day basis. However, this medication is not appropriate for everyone and can be harmful if given to certain individuals.

Consequently, several screening tests must be performed prior to starting treatment to help identify appropriate patients. Gilenya may cause slowing of your heart rate (bradycardia) or an arrhythmia (irregular heart beat). This typically occurs in patients who have a history of heart disease or heart block or in those who are already on medicines that slow the heart rate, such as beta blockers or calcium channel blockers. Tell your physician if you have a history of heart disease. To be cautious, patients must have a baseline EKG performed to verify that they do not have any baseline abnormalities. Gilenya can cause swelling in the back of the eye, known as macular edema. Therefore, patients must complete formal OCT eye testing to screen for macular edema. This is most likely to occur within the first year of treatment and is more common in individuals who are also diabetic. Finally, Gilenya can increase the risk of developing shingles. It is recommended that patients receive the shingles vaccine if they have not previously been vaccinated or if they did not have the chicken pox as a child. This can be tested with a simple blood test called a varicella titer.

Summary of Pre-Testing:

- °   Electrocardiogram
- °   OCT Eye Testing
- °   Varicella Titer
- °   Complete Blood Count
- °   Liver Function Test

Once the pre-testing has been completed and your provider has cleared youth receive the medication, you will be scheduled for your 'first dose observation'. Since the medication can affect your heart rate and rhythm, the first dose of the medication is administered under the supervision of a physician. You will have a repeat EKG done prior to taking the medication. After taking the medication, your blood pressure and heart rate will be monitored hourly for six hours. After six hours, you will have an additional EKG. Assuming everything is normal, you will then continue taking the medication at home like any other medication. If there are concerns in regards to your heart rate or EKG findings, the medical providers will continue to observe you or transfer you to another facility for additional observation or treatment.

Because of lymphocyte and white blood cell suppression, there is a risk of increased infections while taking this medication. This can include serious infections like the rare brain infection PML (progressive multifocal leukoencephalopathy) and cryptococcal infections (fungal infection) but also more common infections like the common cold.[37, 38]

Helpful Hints:

❖ If you plan to start Gilenya, make sure you are not taking blood pressure medications called beta blockers or calcium channel blockers. You will also want to discuss discontinuing any other medications that could interfere with your heart (prolong your QT interval) such as: citalopram, ciprofloxacin, oxybutynin, etc.

❖ Patients experience blurry vision when they develop macular edema. If you have new onset blurry vision while on this medication, contact your provider immediately. Symptoms typically resolve once the medication is discontinued.

❖ OCT testing should be completed every 6 months during the first two years of treatment and annually thereafter.

❖ There is an increased risk of skin cancer and other skin infections for those taking Gilenya. Annual dermatology evaluations are recommended.

❖ Don't skip doses of Gilenya. This could result in needing to repeat your first dose observation. Call your provider if you are wanting to discontinue the medication for any reason.

❖ Take this medication around the same time every day.

❖ If you do experience a decrease in your heart rate after starting the medication, this typically returns to baseline after 4-6 weeks.

❖ If your absolute lymphocyte count drops below 200, your risk for developing serious infections increases. You should discuss alternate therapies with your provider.

TERIFLUNAMIDE (AUBAGIO)

Aubagio is a once a day oral pill that was FDA approved in 2012. It works by preventing the assembly of pyrimidine, a component of DNA, in rapidly dividing cells. This results in fewer abnormal immune cells (T and B cells). Like most MS medications, the exact mechanism in reducing disease activity is not entirely understood. Aubagio has two doses available, 14mg and 7mg.

This medication is tolerated well on a day to day basis. Because the medication targets rapidly dividing cells, there is a small chance of upset stomach and diarrhea. Similarly, it can also cause temporary hair thinning. Although this can be distressing for patients, it will only last for one cycle of hair growth. Generally speaking, this does not warrant changing therapies.

Aubagio can cause liver toxicity although this is rare. You will be required to have monthly lab work for the first six months of treatment to ensure that you do not develop liver damage. Following the first 6 months of labs, routine lab work should be performed every four to six months to evaluate liver enzymes and white blood cell counts.

This medication is not safe to take if you plan to become pregnant. You should have a pregnancy test before you start treatment to confirm you are not pregnant, and it is recommended to be on an effective form of birth control while taking this medication. If you choose to stop Aubagio and would like to conceive, you will need to have your blood checked to evaluate your teriflunomide (Aubagio) blood levels. There is a medication that your provider can prescribe to help eliminate Aubagio from your system at a more rapid pace if desired. Should you become pregnant on this medication, let your healthcare provider know immediately.[39-42]

Helpful Hints:

- ❖ Traces of the medication can stay in your system for up to 2 years.

- ❖ An 11 day course of cholestyramine or activated charcoal can be taken for rapid elimination of Aubagio. You will need to have your blood levels followed to ensure the medication is being eliminated. The lab test is completed at a LabCorp lab and paid for by the drug company (Genzyme).

- ❖ If you experience hair thinning, try taking biotin to help promote hair growth.

- ❖ Like other MS medications, it can also cause reactivation of latent tuberculosis, so a blood test for TB needs to be checked before starting the medicine.

❖ If you experience upset stomach, try taking over the counter medications like Pepto-Bismol and Imodium.

❖ Set a cellphone reminder to help you remember your monthly labs. These are easy to forget a couple of months into treatment.

❖ Take your medication around the same time every day.

DIMETHYL FUMARATE (TECFIDERA)

Dimethyl Fumarate (Tecfidera) is a twice a day oral therapy that was introduced in the spring of 2013. The exact mechanism of action is not entirely understood, however, it is thought to be an anti-inflammatory medication with antioxidant properties. The most distressing side effect related to treatment is upset stomach including nausea, vomiting, bloating, and diarrhea. This is less common if the medication is taken after a meal and tends to improve over time. However, gastrointestinal upset can be idiosyncratic and develop at any time during treatment. Flushing is another commonly reported side effect related to treatment. This can feel like a hot flash, redness, itching, or a rash. Taking the medications with food may also help minimize flushing.

Prior to starting Tecfidera, individuals should have baseline lab work completed to assess their white blood cell count, absolute lymphocyte count, and liver enzyme function. Like many MS medications, Tecfidera can cause a decrease in white blood cell and absolute lymphocyte counts and has been associated with the brain infection PML. Please discuss this with your provider.[43, 44]

Helpful Hints:

❖ Each dose of this medication should be taken as close to 12 hours apart as possible. Using a pill box and a cell phone alarm can be helpful to prevent missing doses.

❖ This medication is not effective if it is not taken twice daily! If you are unable to keep up with multiple doses in a day, let your provider know.

❖ This drug involves a one-week titration where patients take 120mg twice daily for one week before taking the full dose of 240mg twice daily. This is designed to help minimize potential side effects. All patients must reach 240mg twice daily in order for the medication to be fully effective.

❖ This medication has been associated with the rare brain infection PML. To help reduce the risk of this and other serious infections, lab work should be completed every 3-6 months to monitor for low white blood cell counts and lymphocyte counts.

❖ If you experience upset stomach, try taking over the counter medications like Pepto-Bismol and Imodium. Or provider may have additional recommendations so don't be afraid to ask.

❖ Flushing can be ameliorated by taking a baby aspirin (81mg) along with your Tecfidera. Some patients also find taking an antihistamine like Zyrtec or Claritin helpful.

INFUSION THERAPIES

NATALIZUMAB

Natalizumab (Tysabri) is a highly effective monthly IV infusion. It is a monoclonal antibody that targets alpha-4 integrin. It works by making the blood brain barrier 'slippery' thereby preventing immune cells from entering the CNS. It was originally introduced in 2004 but was removed from the market shortly thereafter when several patients exposed to the medication developed the brain infection PML. The medication was reintroduced in 2006 with additional recommendations pertaining to monitoring parameters and concomitant medications. The manufacturer developed a restricted distribution program (TOUCH program) to help improve safety outcomes.

Your risk for PML is dependent on a variety of factors including duration of treatment, exposure to the John Cunningham virus (JC virus), and previous exposure to other immunosuppressive medications. Prior to starting Tysabri, your provider will order a blood test called an anti-JCV antibody index test to see if you have been exposed to the JC virus. This will help your provider advise you of your risk of PML. The JC virus is a common pathogen that is frequently acquired like the flu or the common cold although the mode of transmission has not been well defined. In healthy individuals with a normal immune system, it does not produce an active infection.[45]

Tysabri is generally well tolerated and most patients feel good while on the medication. The most common side effect at the time of the infusion is headaches. Your physician can prescribe medication to treat your headaches if they are not controlled with over the counter medications. Some patients do experience increased infections (urinary tract infections, upper respiratory infections, etc.) while on natalizumab, if this is the case for you, make sure you let your health-care provider know. There are strategies to help reduce the frequency of infections. It is not recommended to receive your infusion while you have an active infection, so you will want to seek treatment for any infections you may develop. Finally, Tysabri should never be stopped suddenly. This puts patients at an increased risk for a relapse, which can often times be severe. If you plan to stop Tysabri, discuss this with your provider, so that you can come up with a plan to transition to another treatment.[46, 47]

Helpful Hints:

❖ You should have your anti-JCV antibody index checked periodically even if it was initially negative. The JC virus is common, and there is a high likelihood that you could seroconvert to JC antibody positive at some point in time.

❖ There are index values available that can help your provider better assess your risk of developing PML.

❖ You will be enrolled in the TOUCH program prior to starting treatment. They will help coordinate finding a certified infusion center near your home where you will receive your monthly infusions.

❖ It is important to be well hydrated at the time of your infusion. Start increasing your water intake the day before your infusion. This will help reduce the risk of potential side effects at the time of your infusion, and it will make it easier for the nurses to gain IV access.

❖ Your body can develop antibodies to the medication, so your provider will periodically check Tysabri antibody tests. If you are found to be positive for Tysabri antibodies, you will need to transition to another medication.

❖ If you experience frequent infections while on this medication, your provider may recommend spacing out the dosing between your infusions or transitioning to another medication. For example, you may receive Tysabri every 6 weeks instead of every 4 weeks.

❖ If there is a delay in receiving your infusion for any reason, let your provider know. It is not safe to miss or skip doses of this medication.

❖ Many patients note improvement in their fatigue and cognitive function after being on the medication for 3-4 months although this is not guaranteed or the primary role of the medication.

ALEMTUZUMAB (LEMTRADA)

Alemtuzumab (Lemtrada) is a promising new therapy for MS patients that offers a unique treatment strategy. It is an infusion medication that patients receive through an IV. It binds to a protein found on T and B cells called CD52. Once the medication binds to these cells, they are subsequently destroyed. Over time, your body slowly regrows new cells and replaces those that were eliminated. The medication is thought to work in two ways. It initially reduces the number of circulating lymphocytes, thus, decreasing the number of T cell and B cells available to enter the CNS. Additionally, it acts by resetting the immune system. Similar to 'control ALT delete' on a PC, once the immune system reboots, it behaves more normally upon return. This is a sustained 'reprograming' of the immune system. The treatment is comprised of two sets of infusions. The first phase of treatment occurs daily for five days and the second is repeated daily for 3 days a year later. Following the second year of infusions, patients have completed the treatment course and should no longer require MS medication.

Due to potential complications, increased infections, and adverse side effects, your provider will order a variety of lab tests to ensure it is safe for you to receive this medication. Baseline labs include: HIV, hepatitis, varicella, TB, pregnancy test, white blood cell count, CD4 count, kidney function, thyroid function, and liver enzyme tests. These assessments must be normal before moving forward with treatment. Some of these tests are required within 30 days of your first infusion.

Serious reactions may occur while you receive your infusion and up to 24 hours (or possibly longer) after you receive the medication. You will complete your infusion at a certified infusion center that has medical personnel trained to manage these reactions. You will be monitored during and after the infusions. If you experience an adverse reaction or develop symptoms concerning for an infusion reaction, your infusion may be discontinued or temporarily paused. Signs of an infusion reaction include rash, itching, swelling of the throat, difficulty breathing, chest pain, or racing heart beats (palpitations). Notify your infusion nurse if you develop any of these symptoms. Your physician will prescribe medications for you to take prior to your Lemtrada infusion to help reduce the risk of developing these symptoms; you will receive IV steroids and likely other pre-medications like diphenhydramine or other anthistamines.

There are also potential long term side effects associated with the medication. In an effort to monitor for potential complications, your healthcare provider will order blood and urine tests every month for 5 years following your first Lemtrada infusion. It is important to have these tests completed even when you are feeling well because they can aid in identify possible problems promptly thereby increasing your chances of better outcomes.

Following exposure to this medication, patients are at increased risk for other autoimmune problems (the immune cells in your body attack other healthy cells in the body). Lemtrada may cause the number of platelets (a cell that helps your blood to clot) in your blood to drop. This is condition called immune thrombocytopenic purpura (ITP), which can cause severe bleeding if left untreated. Call your healthcare provider if you develop easy bruising, bleeding from your gums or nose, or small pink/purple spots on your skin (petechiae). Your physician will be monitoring your platelets with monthly lab work as well.

Lemtrada may also cause a serious kidney problem called anti-glomerular basement membrane disease. This can lead to severe kidney damage and potentially kidney failure if left untreated. Your kidney function will be assessed monthly with blood work and urine tests. Monitor for blood in your urine, swelling in your legs, or high blood pressure.

This medication may increase your risk of certain types of cancers including thyroid cancer, skin cancer, and some blood cancers. It can also cause autoimmune thyroid disease and low blood counts (cytopenias). Once again, the required lab work is intended to capture any abnormalities in blood counts and thyroid function early on so that interventions can be made.[48-50]

Patients on Lemtrada experienced fewer relapses, developed fewer new lesions on their MRIs, and experienced less disability progression, and some individuals even had improvement in their disability![51]

Helpful Hints:

- ❖ After receiving Lemtrada, a large portion of your immune system has been depleted. While you do not have to isolate yourself, it is important to use good hand hygiene and avoid those who are currently ill.

- ❖ Avoid unpasteurized dairy products after receiving Lemtrada and other foods that are known to be contaminated.

- ❖ Taking a variety of antihistamines, steroids, and antacids, prior to your infusion, will likely help minimize possible infusion reactions.

- ❖ Monthly lab work is required for 5 years following your initial infusion even when you are feeling well and asymptomatic. No exceptions.

- ❖ Due to an increased risk of skin cancer, you should have annual dermatology evaluations.

- ❖ This medication is only available through a restricted distribution program called the Lemtrada Risk Evaluation and Mitigation

Strategy (REMS) Program. They will help with monitoring routine lab work.

❖ Lemtrada, like all other MS therapies, is designed to stop new disease activity. Its primary role is not to repair old damage. While many patients do note improvement in their functional ability after receiving this medication, this is not guaranteed and should never be the principal reason for transitioning to this medication.

❖ It is not safe to become pregnant while on this medication. Effective birth control should be used while receiving the medication and for 4 months after the final dose.

❖ Lemtrada can cause an increased risk of infection, so your provider may advise you to take antibiotics or antiviral medications to help prevent infections for a period of time during and following your infusions.

OCRELIZUMAB (Ocrevus)

Ocrelizumab (Ocrevus), an infusion therapy, is the newest approved medication (March 2017) for the management of MS. It has a FDA indication for the treatment of both relapsing forms of MS as well as primary progressive forms of the disease, making it the first of its kind.

It is a monoclonal antibody that works by targeting B cells, more specifically, B cells that express CD20 surface antigens. Cells that have this specific antigen are killed when they come into contact with the medication. Since B cells play an active role in MS disease activity, the medication works by reducing the immune response.

The infusions are administered every six months with the very first infusion being divided in half, in an effort to minimize side effects.

The most common side effects related to treatment are infusion related reactions. As the B cells are dying off, you may experience a rash, itchiness, or difficulty breathing. These side effects are typically avoided when patients are given pre-medications like steroids and antihistamines prior to their infusions.

Overall, the medication has a favorable safety and side effect profile, but it is important to discuss all potential risks with your healthcare provider. Prior to starting the medication, your provider may recommend checking certain blood test to ensure you do not have any active infections such as hepatitis. Like all immunosuppressant treatments, exposure to ocrelizumab may increase your risk of infection or certain cancers.[52] In clinical trials, patients on the medication not only experienced few relapses, fewer new lesions on their MRIs, and less disability progression, but some individuals even had improvement in their disability![53, 54]

Helpful Hints:

❖ You should have baseline laboratory tests completed prior to starting this medication to ensure you do not have any active infections

❖ The first dose is split in half. You will receive one 300mg infusion and then another 300mg infusion two weeks later.

❖ It is important to be well hydrated at the time of your infusion. Start increasing your water intake the day before your infusion. This will help reduce the risk of potential side effects at the time of your infusion, and it will make it easier for the nurses to gain IV access.

❖ Infusion reactions are the most common side effect related to treatment. Discuss possible pre-medications with your provider.

OBTAINING YOUR DISEASE MODIFYING THERAPY

Since MS therapies are highly specialized medications, they are not available at your local pharmacy. They must be shipped to you from a specialty pharmacy. Your insurance provider will be contracted with a specific specialty pharmacy; this will determine which pharmacy distributes your medication.

When starting a new therapy, you and your provider will have you complete a consent form for that given medication. This can be done either electronically or in paper form. This consent form will serve as the prescription for your new therapy. It will then be forwarded to the drug manufacturer along with your insurance information. The drug company will run your insurance benefits and work to obtain insurance approval. After authorization has been received, the prescription then is forwarded to the specialty pharmacy. Once the script has been processed, the pharmacy will contact you directly to schedule shipment of your medication.

Sometimes there is a delay in receiving insurance approval; this can occur for an assortment of reasons and is too variable to discuss in great detail here. However, most drug companies offer 'quick start' programs for those with commercial insurance where they provide free medication to the patient while their provider works to acquire insurance approval. Infusion therapies are typically excluded from 'quick start' programs.

The process is often cumbersome and frustrating for both the patient and provider alike. Delays can be especially frustrating for patients because their providers have emphasized the importance of being on disease modifying therapy with some degree of urgency. So, recognize that while we want you on therapy as soon as possible, it is expected to experience some delay.

Taking the time to understand the process, will help you become a more empowered consumer. Often times, patients have more pull with their insurance companies that providers do. After all, you are their customer, not your physician. Capitalize on this! If you are experiencing delays, contact your insurance company or the drug manufacturer directly.

Helpful Hints:

- ❖ Plan ahead. Allow plenty of time for refills; do not wait until you are almost out of medication before requesting a refill. There are several logistical considerations that go into filling the prescription, all of which take time. A good rule of thumb is to request a refill when you receive the last shipment of your previous script and are out of additional refills.

- ❖ Contact your provider's office directly for refills. Do not rely on the pharmacy to communicate with the doctor's office because oftentimes faxes are not received or miscommunications occur, which leads to frustration and delays.

❖ Most MS medications require prior authorizations before insurance companies will approve them. This is formal documentation that your healthcare provider supplies to the insurer explaining why you need the medication. It can take 7-10 days to gain insurance approval after submission of the appropriate paperwork.

❖ Once you have been stable on a medication, insurance companies will require annual prior authorizations in order for you to continue receiving your medication.

❖ Some insurance companies and specialty pharmacies will only allow patients to receive 30 days of their medication at a time even if their provider has ordered a 90-day supply.

General Considerations Regarding DMTs:

There is not a FDA approved disease modifying therapy approved to take during pregnancy. Generally speaking, there is a 'wash out' period for each medication before it is safe to conceive. The duration of the 'wash out' will vary depending on the medication. Certain medications, like Aubagio or Lemtrada, require more advanced planning. This will be discussed in greater detail in chapter eleven.

Self-administered injections need to be stored in the refrigerator but can be injected at room temperature. Check with your specific medication to see how long it can be left out of the refrigerator.

Set a cell phone alarm to help you remember to take your medication on time. Your medication only works if you take it appropriately. Some find using a bill pox helpful as well.

It is not recommended to receive live vaccines while on most MS therapies. Always consult your provider before receiving a live vaccine if it cannot be avoided.

There is a possibility that you could have a relapse after starting a new medication. This is not considered a treatment failure if it occurs within the first 3-6 months or treatment.

Your provider will likely want to repeat MRIs approximately 6 months after starting a new medication to establish a new baseline for future images to be compared to.

Changing Disease Modifying Therapies

It is normal for patients to try a few medications before they find a treatment that they can both tolerate and that controls their MS disease activity. Only a few patients start on one medication and never have to change therapies. As more effective therapies become available, this trend will likely begin to change. Starting a new medication is typically overwhelming and can feel discouraging, but there are a variety of instances where changing therapies is the most appropriate solution.

Disease progression. Recall that the goal of DMTs is to prevent new disease activity, both clinical relapses (development of new symptoms) and radiological progression (new lesions on MRIs). It takes approximately 3+ months for DMTs to become 100% effective, so after this point if the medication is working, you should not be having new disease activity. If new lesions or clinical symptom arise, this is a definite reason to change strategies and amplify therapy.

Side effects. DMTs are long term treatments and each one has a unique side effect profile. Ideally, when you start a medication, you will be taking it for years to come. That being said, it is unreasonable to expect yourself to take a medication on a long-term basis if you experience significant side effects related to treatment. And the reality is that what you consider significant may or may not be significant for someone else. It is not feasible to stay on a medication long-term if you are not able tolerate the side effects.

Non-compliance. Your MS therapy can only be effective if it is being taken appropriately. Life is busy and it's easy to forget a pill, miss an injection, or delay an infusion, but no medication can have the desired outcome if it is not taken as recommended. Be honest with your provider. If you are missing doses of your medication, you need to switch to something that fits better with your lifestyle. Even the best medication is inadequate if you are not taking it correctly.
Cost. Unfortunately, given the current state of health care, the cost of

medication oftentimes determines its availability. Many insurance companies limit access to specific medication or require 'step therapy,' meaning they require patients to try a number of other medications before they will approve specific therapies. Although providers do their best to choose the most appropriate treatments for their patients regardless of insurance sanctions, sometimes our hands are tied, and we simply cannot get certain medications covered for a given patient. This means that patients have to try an alternative therapy that may not have been the first choice.

Safety concerns. Given the immunosuppressive nature of MS medications and our growing arsenal of therapies, there are a variety of safety ramifications that are associated with each medication. Every time we utilize a treatment, we learn a little more about it and new information becomes available as it is further studied beyond the initial clinical trials. PML is the perfect example. No one was expecting such a strong correlation between PML and Tysabri exposure. Furthermore, most practitioners were not anticipating the risk of PML with exposure to Gilenya and Tecfidera. Alternatively, there may be instances where your perspective changes, and you are no longer comfortable with your given DMT. You may be required to start medication for another disease process that interacts with your MS treatment or you may have elevated liver enzymes while on your treatment and have to transition to something else. As our therapies become more powerful and more successful, they tend to have greater safety concerns, which likely alter your treatment course at one point or another.

Emerging therapies. Thankfully, MS therapies are advancing at a rapid pace. There are currently fifteen FDA approved medications with several others in development and clinical trials, which means there will likely be a time where a superior therapy is introduced to the market. However, newer is not always better and not every patient needs to switch to the latest therapy as soon as it is introduced, but the arrival of new therapies does allow for reconsideration of your treatment strategy.

NEWLY EMERGING TREATMENTS

There are a wealth of newly emerging treatments within the field of MS that are currently being studied. Some represent variations of therapies that are currently available that have mechanisms of action that may be enhanced. Others may just simply be 'generic' versions of existing therapies. Here is a brief list of therapies currently being evaluated, possible indication, and the associated manufacturer.

For Relapsing Forms of MS	For Patients with SPMS	For Myelin Repair	For Progressive MS
ozanimod	siponimod	opicinumab	ibudilast
oral cladribine		rhigm22	
ofatumumab			
monomethyl fumarate			

A QUICK NOTE ABOUT STEM CELL TREATMENTS

There are legitimate stem cell treatment programs for patients with MS and those that are considered 'experimental'. Experimental treatment centers may be found all over the world. Some of our patients have been 'treated' in Costa Rica, Panama, Mexico, China, etc. What patients are truly exposed to (and, where the treatment is obtained from) remains largely unknown. As a result, we do not support such operations.

For stem cell interventions that have been formally evaluated at Universities, understand that these approaches aim to primarily reduce new inflammatory activity and are not geared towards 'repairing' or 'growing' injured myelin or nerves. In addition, the mortality rate associated with such interventions is still considered to be unacceptable by the vast majority of MS specialist.

6

IMAGING

Imaging of the brain and spinal cord is crucial for the diagnosis of MS and for ongoing disease management.[10] It allows us to see the internal manifestations of the disease in addition to the causes for physical signs and symptoms that individuals experience. An assortment of imaging techniques is available today including ultrasound, x-ray, computed tomography (CT), and magnetic resonance imaging (MRI). Each have their own purpose in medicine. MRI scans are how we obtain detailed pictures of the brain and spinal cord, and it is arguably the most useful tool in the diagnosis and surveillance of MS.[55]

MRI scanners use strong magnetic fields and radio frequency waves to create images of specific structures within the body. Images are generated based on the behavior of water in each individual cell. For MS patients, this allows for visualization of the brain and spinal cord in surprisingly clear picture form. It is a very safe test and poses minimal risks to patients.[5]

When viewing a MRI, it's important to note that you are not seeing the entire brain. In addition, only 3 primary planes of view are used. (view section on MRI: Planes of View) Pretend for a second that your brain is a loaf of bread and each picture that we are able to see represents a slice of bread within that loaf. With traditional MRI scans, you are only able to view every other slice of bread. While you do not get to see pictures of the entire brain as a whole, you are able to see large portions of the brain in great detail. There is variability in the thickness of the picture slices depending on the imaging protocol at a given institution, which can impact the quality of your scan. This is referred to as slice thickness. It is the measured thickness of the section of the brain that is being evaluated in each picture. We recommend 3mm slices, meaning each image viewed represents the averaging of 3mm of brain tissue. In between each slice, there is a gap, which is the dead space between each image. If we return to our original analogy, the gap is the "another slice" that we are unable to see. If a lesion was to fall into one of the gaps, we would be unable to capture it, therefore, highlighting the need for small to no gaps between slices. While our technology is not perfect and limitations still exist, imaging the entire brain is now possible at some institutions via 3-dimensional (3D) imaging sequences. By using 3D techniques, not only can full brain coverage be achieved but it may also allow for a new appreciation of the complexity of MS lesions regarding shape and texture. (view section on MS in 3-Dimension)

There are varying types of MRI machines; some are of better quality than others. Like with a camera, the merit of the pictures produced is directly related to the quality of the camera. For MRIs, the picture quality is related to the strength of the magnet and the software used for processing the images. The stronger the magnet used, the sharper the pictures. Commercially available machines utilize 1.5 Tesla and 3.0 Tesla (3T) magnets. When given the choice, always opt for the 3T scanner. When scheduling your MRI ask if they have a 3T machine at their facility. You may also be offered an open MRI, however, these are not recommended for imaging of the brain and spinal cord. The image quality is greatly reduced. However, the open units are needed at times for those who are claustrophobic and for individuals with larger body types.

For healthcare providers, leveraging MRI technology is highly important as MRI relapses (meaning, the development of new plaques or scars) outnumber clinical attacks (i.e. episodes of loss of vision, weakness, etc.) by 10 to 1! Distinct features related to MS injury are observed on your MRI studies. (view section on MRI: Multiple Sclerosis) As MS can affect your optic nerves, brain, and spinal cord, at some point in time, these areas should be evaluated to assess the extent of involvement. Lesions within the infratentorial region (i.e. brainstem, cerebellum, and connecting structures) and spinal cord are more closely associated with disability. (view section on MRI: Brainstem and Spinal Cord).

MRI studies are usually ordered with and without contrast, meaning they take pictures of the brain once then inject contrast dye through an IV, wait a few minutes for the dye to spread through the body, and then take additional pictures. These pictures are referred to as the post contrast images. Gadolinium is the contrast agent used, and it functions as a marker for inflammation. The contrast dye helps identify active lesions. In individuals who do not have any inflammation in their brain, the dye is unable to reach the brain because of a tight barricade called the blood brain barrier. In MS patients, active inflammation allows the dye to leak out of the blood vessel and into the cells causing the MS lesions to appear bright white on the post contrast images.[57] Although post contrast images can be helpful in identifying a current relapse, exposure to contrast dye is not required to see lesions or to evaluate for change over time. For patients with impaired kidney function, who are breast feeding, or with allergies to contrast dye, MRIs can be ordered without contrast.

MRIs are frequently ordered for MS patients to evaluate the brain, optic nerves, and spinal cord.[10, 58] The frequency of each test is dependent on each individual patient and will change with a number of circumstances. Most patients should have imaging of their brain and cervical spinal cord completed at the time of their diagnosis. Even if you meet the latest diagnostic criteria for MS based on your clinical symptoms and brain MRI[15], you should have a MRI of your cervical spine (and, ideally your thoracic spine too) completed as well. This is important, yet often over looked. Baseline imaging of the spinal cord is valuable because the presence of MS lesions in your spinal cord may influence treatment decisions. After starting on disease modifying therapy, you will need to have repeat imaging of your brain completed so that you have a new 'baseline' picture of your brain. This should be completed approximately 6 months after starting your new medication since it takes several months for your DMT to become 100% effective. This scan will be used to compare future MRIs to and will allow you and your provider to know if your medication is preventing new disease activity.[59]

After you have been stable on your therapy, your provider will likely recommend annual MRIs of your brain and possibly your spinal cord (depending on the locations of your previous lesions and reported symptoms). Annual MRIs are used to assess for new or enlarging lesions. Each MRI is compared to the previous scan to evaluate for interval change. It is possible for patients to have new lesions without ever developing new symptoms, and MRIs can help capture those silent changes. Finally, MRIs are used to assess for disease activity when patients are having new or worsening symptoms. The MRIs allow us to see any changes from the prior study, and the post contrast images identify any current disease activity. As previously discussed, when there is active demyelination, the contrast dye is able to leak into the brain in the areas of inflammation. This is known as blood brain barrier compromise. This makes the active lesions appear bright white on the MRI pictures. You may hear your provider refer to this as contrast enhancement.[60] (view section on MRI: Contrast Enhancement)

MRIs are one of the key measures used for monitoring for disease progression. New lesions identified on MRIs generally indicate evidence of disease activity and/or evolution. However, there are a few instances in which new changes are related to advancing age or other health conditions and not indicative of MS disease activity. Examples include high blood pressure, migraines, diabetes, or smoking.[60] If new MS lesions are identified on your imaging studies, this suggests that your DMT may not be providing the protection that it should. As we discussed in the last chapter, this is when you should discuss changing your disease modifying therapy with your provider.

Helpful Hints:

❖ MRIs are used for diagnosis, surveillance, or to assess for new disease activity when having symptoms.

❖ Not all MRIs are equal. Image quality depends on the quality of the MRI magnet. MRIs should be completed on at least a 1.5T magnet and ideally should be completed on a 3T magnet if possible.

❖ There are 'open MRIs' for patients who are claustrophobic, while these may be sufficient for some studies, this will not provide high quality images of the brain or spinal cord. You need to have a 'closed MRI.'

❖ If you are claustrophobic, your provider can prescribe MRI sedation. You will need someone to drive you to and from your appointment.

❖ Every time you have a MRI, request a copy of the CD for your personal record. You will need to take these with you to your neurologist appointments for their review.

❖ It is possible for patients to have new lesions without ever developing new symptoms. This is why annual MRIs are important. They can help capture silent changes.

❖ Contrast can be helpful but is not necessary if you have an allergy or impaired kidney function.

❖ If you are allergic to contrast dye, your provider may choose pre-treat with Benadryl and steroids to help prevent an allergic reaction instead of recommending a non-contrast study.

❖ Some medical devices are not MRI compatible. Please let your provider know if you have any implanted devices or hardware.

❖ New MS lesions can enhance on MRI for several weeks.

❖ There are often changes identified on MRI that are related to aging or other health conditions and are not necessarily indicative of MS although they can resemble MS lesions

❖ Have imaging of the cervical spine completed when you are diagnosed. Since disease activity in the spinal cord correlates with more aggressive disease, and it can be predictive of future outcomes, it's critical information to have.

❖ Keep a personal copy of every MRI you complete.

❖ Take a copy of your recent MRI and the radiologist's report to your office visit every time you go.

❖ The spinal cord terminates at the level of the lumbar spine, so the lumbar spine is not routinely imaged in the evaluation of multiple sclerosis. This test may be ordered to evaluate specific symptoms.

For more comprehensive information regarding MRI data in MS, please refer to our online resource. (search Understanding MRI: MS in the App Store or Google Play)

MRI: PLANES OF VIEW

There are only 3 primary planes of view that we are able see from your MRI study. The first (A), is an axial view. The second (B), is a coronal or face on view. Lastly (C), a sagittal view is available. By using these planes of view, healthcare providers are able to determine the size and location of any lesions present and verify that the observed changes are the result of injury from MS.

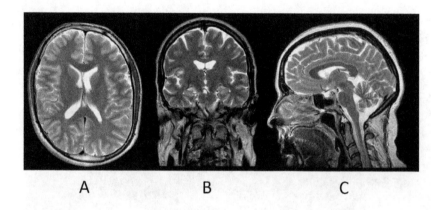

A   B   C

MS IN 3-DIMENSION

We did something that no one has ever done before and developed a new technique to study the 3-dimensional characteristics of brain lesions resulting from MS. By evaluating MS lesions in this way, we identified dynamic shapes and textures (right panel). The study of the different shapes and textures may allow for the determination of lesion age while providing insights into the degree of injury present. These data may also inform on risk for future disability (visit **www.ardireo.com** for more information)

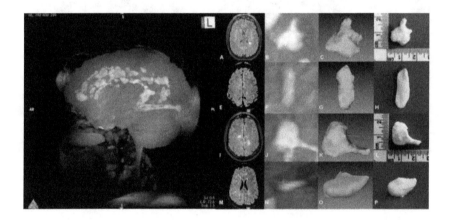

MRI: MULTIPLE SCLEROSIS

The diagnosis of MS is made based on an individual's clinical experience, findings on neurological examination, laboratory studies, and MRI features. We ensure that there is not a better explanation for your symptoms and MRI findings. The MRI findings (circled in yellow), also referred to as lesions, bright spots, T2-hyperintensities, plaques, etc., result from the immune system inaccurately causing harm to normal tissue. More recent science has allowed us to appreciate how complex each of these lesions are in shape and texture.

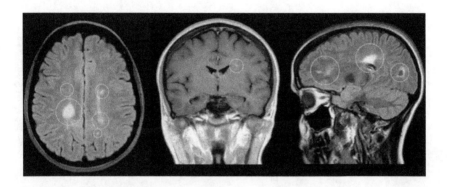

Below is an image of a single MS lesion revealing its true shape and surface complexity.

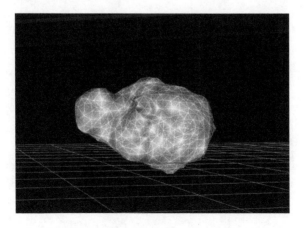

MRI: BRAINSTEM AND SPINAL CORD REGIONS

Multiple sclerosis lesions may occur within the optic nerves, brain, infratentorial region (i.e. brainstem, cerebellum, and connecting structures), and the spinal cord. A. MRI in sagittal plane (side profile view) demonstrating MS lesions within the brainstem and cervical spinal cord (white arrows). B. MS lesions within the thoracic spinal cord region (yellow arrows). C. MRI in cross-section showing a cervical spinal cord lesion (white arrow). D. MS lesion involving the cerebellum (white arrow).

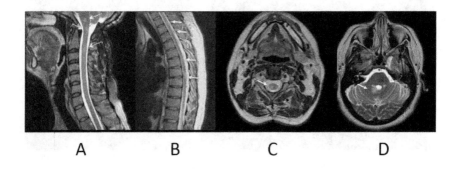

A   B   C   D

MRI: CONTRAST ENHANCEMENT

Gadolinium (or, contrast) is frequently used with MRI studies to assess for the presence of new MS lesions (or, to identify new enlargement of existing lesions). In the left panel, a pre-contrast MRI is shown highlighting a MS lesion. Following the administration of contrast, enhancement (open ring) of that lesion can be seen (right panel). Note that there is also mild enhancement present in the brainstem (red ring).

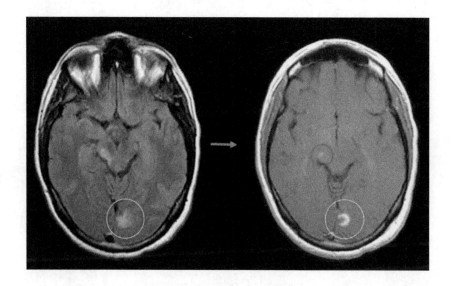

7

IT'S ALL RIGHT HERE

What is a MS relapse?

A relapse is often referred to as an MS attack, exacerbation, or flare. Periodic relapses are a distinguishing feature of the disease. It is the clinical manifestation of active inflammation and demyelination within the brain and/or spinal cord, which results in symptomatic deterioration. Simply put, a relapse involves the development of new or worsening symptoms that last more than 24 hours. In order to qualify as a true relapse, these symptoms cannot be attributed to other factors such as increased stress, infection, or fatigue. Typically, symptoms occur unexpectedly and increase in intensity over hours to days. Patients experience varying degrees of symptomatic recovery over the course of weeks to months following symptom onset.[2, 61, 62]

Signs of a MS Relapse
New numbness/tingling of the face, trunk, or extremities
Weakness of the arms or legs
New walking or balance difficulties
New dizziness
New bladder or bowel difficulties

Helpful Hints:

❖ If you believe you may be having a relapse, contact your provider.

❖ In the event that you have new symptoms, you will likely be asked to be evaluated in clinic by one of your providers.

❖ You may also be asked to complete lab work or imaging prior to your appointment.

❖ Always use your best judgement, if you feel as if your symptoms are escalating quickly or are of an urgent nature, please go to the Emergency Room.

Treating a Relapse

It is not necessary to treat every new symptom medically, and generally speaking, many symptoms are inappropriately identified as a relapse and subsequently treated within the community. Even for a true relapse, medical intervention is not required.[61] Following a relapse, some degree of biological recovery is expected, so it is difficult to know how much improvement is specifically related to prescribed therapies versus the body's own ability to heal itself. The most significant recovery occurs within the first 6 months following symptom onset. Injuries sustained during a relapse may resolve entirely but often times there is some degree of permanent damage. Data are limited in regards to the long-term benefits of treating exacerbations although intuitively one would think there are advantages to reducing the active inflammation that is present during a relapse. The treatment goal for an acute relapse is to improve your quality of life by lessening symptoms and shortening the duration of your recovery following a relapse. Currently, the scientific data suggests that steroid treatment for an exacerbation does not change long-term outcomes. This highlights the importance of treatment to prevent relapses from every occurring!

There are several different treatment options available for relapses. Response to these interventions can be quite variable depending on the patient and not all patients respond to each agent.[63]

Steroid Side Effects[61]

Swelling of the arms and/or legs

Increased appetite and weight gain

Upset stomach/stomach ulcers

Elevated blood sugar levels

Sleep disturbance

High blood pressure

Joint pain

Mood changes

Glucocorticosteroids

Management with high dose corticosteroids is the mainstay of treatment, which can be given either intravenously (IV) or orally. Treatments with methylprednisolone (Solumedrol), dexamethasone (Decadron), or prednisone are commonly prescribed. The existing scientific data suggests that steroids in IV or oral form are similar in their effectiveness in providing symptom relief.[64] High dose steroids have both anti-inflammatory and immunosuppressive properties that help to reduce active inflammation. The medication is typically taken for 3-5 days depending on your provider's preference and the nature of your symptoms.[61, 65] Longer treatment durations are pursued when symptoms are severe. A lower probability of symptom recurrence exists with longer treatment durations. Typically, initial improvements occur within the first week of exposure to the medication and continue to occur for weeks following treatment.[66, 67] As with any therapy, steroids are not without their own side effects, and unfortunately, there are both immediate and long term consequences associated with steroid exposure.

Long Term Consequences of Steroid Exposure

Increased risk of osteoporosis - thinning of bones, which can make one more susceptible to fractures

Increased risk of cataracts

Risk of avascular necrosis- tiny fractures occur in a bone over time due to reduced blood supply. Ultimately, the bone collapses. This notoriously occurs in the hip

Weight gain

Helpful Hints:

- ❖ Always take oral steroids with a full meal to help prevent an upset stomach

- ❖ Corticosteroids increase acid secretion in your stomach. When receiving steroids, either orally or IV, take an antacid medication such as esomeprazole. Continue the antacid for 30 days following the steroids.

- ❖ If you experience fluid retention, try decreasing your sodium intake and elevating legs when possible.

- ❖ Since steroids can cause sleep disturbance, it is best to take the medication in the morning. Never take steroids after lunchtime.

❖ Diabetics should monitor their blood sugar levels closely and may require insulin while on steroids.

AcTHar Gel

For patients who do not tolerate steroids or who have a suboptimal response, AcTHar Gel is another treatment option. AcTHar is a purified formulation of the hormone adrenocorticotropin (ACTH). It works by stimulating the body to produce its own steroid hormones, which in turn, help to reduce inflammation. It is also thought that AcTHar may affect the function of T cells and B cells as well, but this is not fully understood. The medication comes in a gel form that is injected under the skin (SQ) or into the muscle (IM) once daily for 5-10 days.[8, 63, 68]

This is an effective treatment option that tends to have fewer side effects compared to steroids; however, it is unknown if this treatment is as effective as steroids for MS exacerbations as there are no available prior study data. It is a great option for patients who have significant side effects with high dose steroid or who are unable to take steroids. AcTHar may be considered for those with poorly controlled diabetes because it does not cause elevated blood sugar levels to the same degree as high dose steroids. While the medication is effective and well tolerated, it can be difficult to obtain insurance approve due to the cost of the medication, which often times leads to treatment delays.[63, 69]

Helpful Hints:

❖ AcTHar is a great option for those who cannot tolerate high dose oral or IV steroids.

❖ It is an injectable therapy. Injection training is available through the drug company.

❖ Having a documented adverse reaction to corticosteroids, will help with obtaining insurance approval.

Plasmapheresis

Plasmapheresis is a procedure also known as plasma exchange or PLEX. It is can be considered in the treatment of MS relapses when there are persistent deficits despite other interventions like steroids or AcTHar. Plasma exchange is a process that filters a portion of the blood called plasma. Once the plasma has been removed, it is replaced with the donor plasma or other replacement fluid. The premise of treatment is that the removal of certain substances like antibodies and other immune cells may limit inflammation and help reverse symptoms.[1, 70]

Plasma exchange can be completed in the hospital or in an outpatient clinic depending on your provider's resources. It is a relatively non- invasive procedure that is achieved by placing a catheter in a large vein that can facilitate large volumes of blood flow. The duration of treatment is patient and provider specific but typically 5-7 treatments occur over the course of a couple weeks.

Plasma exchange is a second-line treatment that is aimed at improving patient function and addressing persistent symptoms.[70]

Helpful Hints:

❖ PLEX is a blood purification technique for the removal of plasma, which houses cells that are contributing to MS disease activity.

❖ Successful treatment requires reliable venous access

❖ Treatment duration is typically based on patient response

Intravenous Immunoglobulin (IVIg)

Intravenous immunoglobulin (IVIg) was previously used to treat MS exacerbations more rigorously approximately 10 years ago. The current use of this agent is limited to patients who have breakthrough disease after receiving high-dose steroid treatment and PLEX or if patients are found to be intolerant to or have refractory disease after receiving steroids. This treatment is typically used following PLEX to prevent these proteins from being filtered out. At present, the use of IVIg is more robust as a relapse preventative agent in the post-partum period as prior scientific data failed to demonstrate a benefit in the treatment of acute optic neuritis.[71]

Take Home Messages:

- ❖ A relapse involves the development of new or worsening symptoms that last more than 24 hours.

- ❖ It is not necessary to treat every symptomatic complaint with steroids.

- ❖ These treatments aim to provide improvement of acute symptoms. They are not intended to address long standing complaints.

- ❖ Acute treatment modalities reduce new deficits but do not effect long-term disease activity.

- ❖ We are unsure if the treatment of acute relapses with steroids improves long term outcomes, therefore, the prevention of **relapses is key!**

- ❖ In the future, software (yes, software!) may be prescribed to patients with MS to assess if an exacerbation is present. To experience *our* prototype for the future of MS care, additional information may **be found here.** (search MS Relapse Tool in the App Store or Google Play).

8

ADJUNCT THERAPIES AND COMPLEMENTARY MEDICINE

For MS patients, there are a variety of DMT medications aimed at preventing new disease activity. However, we are more limited when it comes to therapies that provide functional benefit to patients. This chapter outlines the few available therapies that we do have, which you may find helpful in addressing more functional concerns such as walking and day-to-day activities. Specific symptomatic medications will be addressed separately in a later chapter.

Walking difficulties are one of the most common concerns for MS patients. Being able to maintain one's mobility, is key to preserving their independence. In order to do so, one must be able to navigate their home and work place safely. When it comes to mobility, difficulty can arise in a variety of settings. Some patients may have trouble climbing stairs or walking long distances while others may have trouble lifting their feet with regular walking. Ampyra (dalfampridine) is a prescription medicine that is used to help improve walking (gait) in MS patients. It has been shown to increase walking speed and quality of gait.[72]

To understand how this medication works, one must understand how communication occurs along a nerve. Information is carried from the brain to the body via electrical impulses. Abrupt changes in electrical charges prompt waves of electrical stimuli that travel along from one neuron to the next. This is called polarization and occurs as a result of the influx and efflux of charged molecules (ions) in and out of the neuron. Sodium and potassium are two principal ions involved. The signal is able to travel down the nerve axon due to differences in electrical charge inside and outside of the cell brought about by sodium and potassium. At rest, the nerve cell is negatively charged on the inside while the outside of the cell is positively charged. The cell maintains its negative charge by pumping sodium out of the cell and forcing potassium inside.[73, 74]

When the nerve becomes activated, there is an abrupt change in the voltage across the cell wall. As a nerve is stimulated, protein channels open up allowing a rapid influx of sodium ions, thus, making the cell positively charged. This allows the information to be passed along to the neighboring nerve cell. Once this has occurred, the cell then works to pump the sodium back out of the cell and potassium back inside. This process is called repolarization, and it prepares the cell to be activated again. Myelin (the insulation around the nerve cell) allows for more rapid transmission of signals along the nerve through a process called salutatory conduction. In addition to the increasing speed of travel down a nerve, the myelin also allows the body to conserve energy by limiting the influx and efflux of ions that would otherwise be required.[73, 74] For MS patients, the transmission of electrical impulses is impaired due to the damaged myelin and nerves.

Ampyra works by blocking potassium channels thereby improving the conduction of signals in damaged cells.[72] Ampyra is a time released tablet that is taken orally every 12 hours. It can take anywhere from a few days up to 6 weeks for patients to notice an improvement in their walking ability, and not every patient notes improvement after being on treatment. There are also differing levels of response amongst patients. Some individuals have a dramatic response to treatment while other do notice modest improvement. Therefore, it is important to monitor your walking before and after starting therapy to gauge your response. Your provider will likely monitor your response to treatment with a timed 25-foot walk. They will assess how long it take you to walk 25 feet both before and after treatment to evaluate for improvement.[75] Many patients also note improvement in their fatigue and heat intolerance while on this medication although these are not the primary reasons for starting the medication (approved indications).

Ampyra is not safe to take for those who have a history of seizure events. Due to the risk of having a seizure, the medication should also be taken exactly as prescribed. The dose strength or frequency should never be increased as this will put you at an increased risk of seizures.[75]

This medication should also be avoided in those with kidney disease. Your provider will check your serum creatinine (blood test) to test your kidney function prior to starting treatment. This is important because impaired kidney function will increase your risk of seizures.[75]

Helpful Hints:

❖ Not everyone responds to this medication

❖ The medication is taken 10mg every 12 hours

❖ Do not take more than directed. EVER! More is not better even if you have a great response to the medication

❖ If you miss a dose, skip it and get back on schedule with the next one

❖ The medication is time released, so do not cut it in half or crush it unless you have been specifically instructed to do so by your provider.

❖ Low dose naltrexone (LDN) is a medication that is used off label as an adjunct treatment for MS patients. Naltrexone is an opioid antagonist and thus, blocks opioid receptors. It is approved to treat opioid and alcohol dependence. However, it is used at lower doses in MS patients and other autoimmune diseases because it is thought to increase natural endorphins and potentially exert positive effects on the immune system.[76]

❖ LDN should never be used in place of DMTs, but it can be beneficial for symptom management. Patients often find it helpful for pain, spasticity, fatigue, depression, and sleep.[76, 77] It is a compounded medication, so it must be made at a compounding pharmacy. Many compounding pharmacies ship medication if there is not one near your home. The medication is generally taken at bedtime and is tolerated well overall.

Complementary and Alternative Medicine Strategies

Individuals seek complementary and alternative medicine for a variety of reasons. One may be looking for symptomatic relief while another may be hoping to slow disease progression. Regardless of the desired outcome, it is important to note that the safety and efficacy of many complementary and alternative therapies have not been formally established. There are limited scientific studies available for us to draw adequate conclusions. Therefore, it is important to keep your provider up-to-date on the therapies or treatment strategies you are pursuing.

Acupuncture

Acupuncture has been a fundamental component of Chinese medicine, and there are a wide variety of practices and different philosophies used depending on the practitioner. In traditional Chinese medicine, physical ailments occur as a result of an imbalance in energy flow throughout the body. Small, flexible needles are inserted into specific pressure points in an effort to alter this flow of energy. There are several hundred acupressure points that can be utilized. Many patients find acupuncture helpful for management of pain, muscle spasms, fatigue, headaches, and sleep disturbances. It typically takes several rounds of treatment for patients to experience notable benefit. While it may be helpful for certain symptoms, acupuncture should not be used as a means for managing disease progression and should never take the place of a FDA approved disease modifying therapy.[77, 78]

Reflexology

Reflexology therapy is a pressure technique that is customarily focused on the feet or hands. This treatment is centered around the belief that there are specific regions and reflexes in the hands and feet that correlate to other body systems. The stimulation of these specific zones is thought to facilitate circulation and relaxation thereby enabling the body to excrete toxins and promoting relaxation.[79]

Cannabis

Symptomatic management with cannabis is a growing area of interest among patients as medicinal use is becoming more widely accepted. In terms of MS, it's utility is generally geared towards the treatment of pain and muscle spasms. There are two key components of cannabis: δ-9-tetrahydrocannabinol (THC) and cannabidiol (CBD). THC is the main psychotropic agent, meaning it can alter brain function and affect one's level of consciousness and mood. CBD, on the other hand, is not psychoactive and makes up a large component of the plant.[80] There have been several clinical trials that have assessed the efficacy of using varying combinations of THC and CBD to treat spasticity. While patients reported improvement in their symptoms, objective measures, like a timed walk and physical exam, did not show clear improvement following treatment.[77, 81] The long-term health effects associated with cannabis use are not well established at this point, and one must consider your state's legal stance when considering the use of medical marijuana.

Supplements

Do I need to check with my provider before purchasing or starting a new supplement?

It is important to tell all of your medical providers if you plan to start taking a new supplement, not just your neurologist. Make sure you discuss what you are taking at every visit so that your medical record can be updated accordingly. Certain supplements may interfere with prescription medications. Some supplements may need dose adjustments and others may need to be avoided entirely.

Can supplements be used to treat my MS in place of traditional medication?

There is not clear evidence to support the use of supplements as a means for regulating MS disease activity. Some supplements may be helpful for treating specific symptoms like fatigue, sleep disturbances, or headaches.

N-acetyl-glucosamine is a supplement that is derived from glucose, a form of sugar. It has been used in the treatment of autoimmune diseases because it is thought to inhibit T cell function.[82] The great thing about N-acetyl-glucosamine is that it is easily accessible and relatively inexpensive form of treatment. However, data are limited, and it should not replace the use of a FDA approved MS treatment.

Turmeric is an over the counter supplement from the ginger family. Curcumin is the active compound found in turmeric, which has anti-inflammatory and antioxidant properties. There are claims that it also has neuroprotective effects, however, this has not been well studied.[83]

Biotin (vitamin B7) has been given much attention in recent years for its potential role in myelin repair. At high doses (10 times that of normal dosing recommendations), biotin may help slow symptom progression and possibly lead to improvement in functional status.[84, 85] It is important to mention that exposure to biotin may invalidate thyroid function and cardiac enzyme test results.[86]

Cranberry supplements may be considered a natural remedy for preventing urinary tract infections. When taken regularly with ample amounts of water, it may aid in preventing infections. It is important to note, however, that it will not treat current infections.[77, 87] If an active infection is suspected, please reach out to your provider. If left untreated, it could lead to serious complications. Another option for prevention of urinary tract infections is D-mannose. This agent is thought to prevent the binding of bacteria to the bladder wall. A previous randomized study demonstrated an effect similar to a common antimicrobial treatment used in preventing infections, nitrofurantoin (Macrobid).[86]

9

DIET

A number of emerging theories have linked the effects of environmental exposures and lifestyle choices to the development of MS, disease activity, and disease progression.[3, 5, 89-92] Like we have mentioned before, lifestyle changes offer a secondary prevention strategy in addition to traditional disease modifying therapies. Modifiable risk factors like diet, exercise, and smoking are a few target areas for intervention. These are elements in which patients have direct control and have the opportunity to be an active participant in their own self-management. Your overall health greatly impacts your neurological health! This can't be emphasized enough.

Good nutrition is an important part of wellness for anyone, but this especially holds true for those with chronic disease. Measuring the outcomes of diet and MS symptoms is arduous, thus, data are limited. This is a challenging area to study due to multiple variables that are difficult to regulate in formal clinical trials. Ultimately, no single diet will be a miracle cure for MS, but food choices do matter. There is increasing evidence that suggest our typical 'Western diet' influences our body's immune response.[92]

Generally speaking, we are an overfed and undernourished culture where convenience has become the primary focus when it comes to food. Fast and easy food choices have trumped healthy and fresh alternatives. The standard American diet is characterized by an overabundance of saturated fats, omega-6 fatty acids, refined sugar, grains, and salt. There is science behind how these ingredients are added to our foods. There are scientists whose primary role is to make processed foods even more tasty and attractive to consumers. And they are doing an excellent job; in 2014, it was reported that Americans spent $117 billion on fast food alone![93]

When considering our food intake or 'diet,' nutrient content should be our main focus. If we are eating real, fresh, whole foods, the remaining details become less important.

Understanding the basic composition of food is essential. Food is comprised of macro and micronutrients, both of which are necessary for our bodies to function properly. Macronutrients include protein, carbohydrates, and fat. These are energy yielding nutrients that provide calories for our bodies to convert to mechanical energy. Micronutrients include vitamins and minerals; they do not generate energy but help regulate the body's functions.[94] It is always best to get these nutrients from fresh fruits, vegetables, and lean proteins. Our lifestyles should be centered around natural, raw, whole foods not simply supplemented with the occasional fruit and vegetable.

The abundance of food within our culture has led to overconsumption and weight gain. We have learned to treat our bodies like a garbage receptacle, eating anything that is available. We have been conditioned to eat for stimulation instead of nourishment. As a society, we eat foods that are highly processed, easy to obtain, and highly addictive. Processed foods are detrimental to our health for a variety of reasons; they are overflowing with refined sugars and modified fats, which are known to contribute to a variety of health consequences including obesity, heart disease, and diabetes.[95] There is increasing evidence to suggest that dietary habits can affect autoimmune diseases, like MS, in various ways.[96, 97] Highly processed foods are more difficult for the body to digest and may alter the gut microbiome (healthy bacteria within the intestines), which in turn, negatively effects one's immune system.[92, 95] On the other hand, plant based foods like fruits and vegetables, have anti-inflammatory potential and encourage the growth of healthy bacteria within the intestines.[98, 99] Supplementing a healthful diet with high quality probiotics can also help populate your digestive system with beneficial bacteria.[95]

There are several specific diets that have gained popularity within the MS community over the past decade, however, there is limited evidence as to how these specific protocols actually affect patient outcomes and disease course. Often times, diet protocols are highly regimented and not very practical for most people. When it comes to diet, quality of life is an important factor for sustainable, long-term change. Do not implement drastic interventions that are going to be distressing for you or your family.

Outlined below are a few specific food types that have gained popularity for their potential influence on daily symptoms and/or the immune system.

Gluten- Some data suggests that there is a higher incidence of gluten intolerance in MS patients when compared to the general population.[100, 101] In animal models, gluten can stimulate inflammation and alter the gut microbiota.[92, 95] Therefore, patients may benefit from eliminating or minimizing gluten intake. A gluten free diet means avoiding wheat, rye, barley, and triticale foods (and their derivatives).

Dairy - In one study, MS patients were found to have a greater immune response to casein (one of the main proteins found in milk and dairy products) when compared to healthy controls.[101] Alternatively, another protein, butyrophilin, which is found in milk fat has been shown to have similar properties to an autoantigen found in MS.[92, 102] A dairy free diet may be beneficial and involves avoiding foods made from milk; this includes most yogurt, butter, and cheese.

Some suggest following an "autoimmune diet" in which all grains, nuts, beans/legumes, seeds, eggs, dairy, and nightshade vegetables are avoided along with alcohol, artificial sweeteners, and food additives. This is based on the premise that these foods increase inflammation. Data are inadequate as to whether or not these restrictions are beneficial. Additionally, consuming a diet high in animal products, puts individuals at risk for a variety of other diseases like diabetes and cardiovascular disease.

Vitamin D - Low levels may increase the risk of MS and may be related to an increased risk of relapse.[3] However, newly emerging data suggests that body mass index may be a more important risk factor than vitamin D status.

Sodium - Animal studies suggest that high dietary salt intake may increase inflammation and may be a risk factor for the development of autoimmune disease.[103-105] However, recent data suggest that high sodium diets are not associated with a more aggressive MS disease course.[106] Data are limited and more information is need before formal recommendations can be made. However, limiting sodium intake to less than 1,500 mg per day is ideal for overall heart health.[107]

Miscellaneous foods - There are other foods that you may consider avoiding although their direct impact on MS is not well defined. These include aspartame, caffeine, and alcohol to name a few. Excessive amounts of caffeine can interfere with your sleep/wake cycle and can cause bladder irritation. Excess alcohol can compound gait and balance difficulties.

Certain supplements like spirulina, Echinacea, and garlic should be avoided as they may have immunostimulating effects, which in theory could negatively affect MS disease activity.[108-110] Check the labels of your protein powders and drink mixes. Anything that is marketed as an 'immune booster' should be avoided.

When it comes to diet, it is important to remember that no single food ever operates in isolation. Each nutrient we consume interacts, either synergistically or in conflict, with everything else we ingest. Therefore, a healthful diet rich in fruits and vegetables is likely more beneficial than eliminating specific foods or adding multiple supplements.

The gut microbiome also plays a critical role in immune function. There are up to 1,000 difference bacterial species that work to keep us healthy. Most of the bacteria present in the human gut are the phyla Bacteroidetes and Firmicutes, and the ratio between the two is largely determined by longstanding dietary patterns.[97, 111, 112] A link has been identified between MS and the gut microbiome, making it an area of great interest.[113]

The human gut is initially colonized during infancy and is constantly being recolonized throughout adulthood. The changes that occur throughout one's life span are multifactorial; diet, stress, and medication exposure are a few contributing factors.[97, 114, 115] When the optimal balance between bacterial species is disrupted, there are accompanying shifts in regards to inflammation and immune function.[111, 116] Healthy gut bacteria support the presence of regulatory T-cells, which work to encourage balance within our immune system. These same healthy bacteria also limit the presence of pro-inflammatory Th17 cells.[117] Generally speaking, a higher ratio of Firmicutes to Bacteroidetes is associated with inflammatory and auto-immune disease.[118] Through dietary practices, we have the opportunity to adjust the composition of this complex microbial community to a more favorable ratio of Bacteroidetes to Firmicutes. Plant based diets rich in complex carbohydrates promote colonization of Bacteroidetes while a 'Western diet' high in proteins, animal fat, and refined sugars and grains, promotes a predominance of Firmicutes.[97, 119]

Aside from influencing the population of bacteria in the gut, our diet may also directly affect how our bodies process the food we consume.[92, 120] More favorable pathways of energy metabolism are stimulated by a low-calorie diet rich in fruits, vegetables, fiber, and omega-3 fatty acids. On the other hand, the typical high calorie 'Western diet' can activate a less favorable, more inflammatory pathway.[92] A link has been established between high-fat diets and increased inflammation, and it has been suggested that the consumption of animal based fat may be associated with MS.[121, 122]

Obesity, like other comorbid diseases, also impacts MS. Fat tissue is not inert; it secretes pro-inflammatory cells. Therefore, when overabundant, it promotes low-grade, systemic inflammation, which highlights our need to maintain a healthy weight.[123, 124] However, maintaining a healthy weight can be particularly troublesome for MS patients; the disadvantage is multifactorial. Every extra pound adds strain to (in many cases) already weak muscles making walking, standing, or transferring extra challenging. Secondly, it can be more difficult for individuals with MS to lose excess weight because they are limited in their ability to exercise due to heat sensitivity, muscle weakness, pain, or balance difficulties. Weight gain can also contribute to increased fatigue, depression, and cardiovascular risk factors.

If you are looking to make dietary changes, we recommend adopting a whole-food, plant based diet. This pattern of eating eliminates the foods that are most likely to cause inflammation and immune response while also promoting a healthy gut microbiome. Plants are rich in nutrients and a natural source of antioxidants and fiber. They also contain polyphenols, which have anti- inflammatory and immunomodulatory effects.[125-127]

Additionally, a whole-food, plant based diet rich in fruits, vegetables, tubers, whole grains, and legumes, can produce rapid, quantifiable change in a number of health measures. In fact, it has been recommended for the prevention and treatment of many common chronic diseases like heart disease, diabetes, and some forms of cancer, all of which can occur alongside MS. [128-130]

We have the power to change our health outcomes both individually and collectively with our food choices. Every time we purchase food, we support the system that created it. As consumers, we have the opportunity to promote access to whole, healthy foods!

It may take several months after eliminating specific food groups from your diet to notice a change in how you feel, so don't get discouraged. Try to stick with it for at least 90 days. Focus on one item at a time; pick what is easiest for you to give up and start by limiting that component first. Once you have mastered one food group, move on to the next. Take your time; you want to produce sustainable change. While a whole-food, plant based diet is most ideal, it does not have to be all or nothing. There is still benefit in making small changes. So, if making extensive changes all at once is overwhelming for you, start by eliminating dairy products and limiting meat consumption to 2-3 days a week. Have your primary focus be increasing fruit and vegetable consumption. Once you have mastered that, you can consider making additional changes.

Dietary changes and FDA approved disease modifying therapies work synergistically to attain the best possible outcomes. Take some time to reflect on your current dietary habits because food choices do matter. As you contemplate making positive lifestyle changes, here are some general principles to consider.

A Healthful Diet Is:

Sufficient - your diet must provide adequate energy, nutrients, fiber, water, and vitamins to support your health.

Moderate - a healthy diet contains the appropriate quantity of foods to maintain a healthy weight.

Balanced - your diet should consist of the appropriate combination of foods to provide a suitable balance of nutrients.

Varied - a healthy diet consists of foods from a variety of food groups.

Will a specific diet cure my MS?

No single diet will cure MS. A balanced, healthful diet that is rich in fruits and vegetables should be your primary goal.

Is there a way to identify which foods my body reacts to?

Yes, there is commercial food allergy testing available that assess your degree of sensitivity to a variety of different foods. Unfortunately, insurance companies typically do not cover the cost of these tests. Speak with your healthcare provider to see if this is appropriate for you.

What is a plant based diet?

A whole-food, plant based diet is centered around consuming primarily fruits, vegetables, and unrefined whole grains. Animal products like meat (beef, chicken, pork, fish, etc.) eggs, and dairy are avoided. All oils and processed foods such as white flour, sugar, and 'convenience foods' should also be limited.

Interested in a transition to a plant based diet? If so, be sure to check out our resource as it contains a wealth of information including meal planning strategies, recipes, and the ability for you to log your own designed meals! (search Plant Process in the App Store or Google Play)

Can I get enough protein from a plant-based diet?

Yes, there is adequate protein in a variety of plant-based foods including beans, nut, seeds, soy, vegetables, and whole grains. The CDC's most recent Dietary Guidelines recommended a daily intake or 46 grams and 56 grams of protein for adult women and men, respectively. Over half of the US population exceeds this recommendation.[131]

This recommended target is easily achievable with a plant based diet.

- ° ½ cup spinach 3 grams

- ° ½ cup black beans 8 grams

- ° 1 Tb peanut butter 7 grams

- ° ½ cup lentils 9 grams

- ° ½ cup quinoa 4 grams

- ° 1 ounce almonds 6 grams

Can I get all the nutrients I need from a plant- based diet?

Plants have the highest quality nutrients of all foods. Have you ever stopped to think how animal products provide nutrients at all? They acquire them from the plants they consume. With a plant based diet, you are going straight to the source. With the exception of vitamin B12, you can attain all the necessary nutrients from plants. Many foods like whole grain cereal, nutritional yeast, and nut milks are fortified with B12. Alternatively, you can supplement with an over the counter supplement.

Is it bad to eat so many carbs on a plant- based diet?

No, the movement to limit carbohydrates is the result of trendy diets like the Atkins diet, South Beach diet, and most recently, the paleo diet. Carbohydrates are our body's primary energy source. That being said, our carbohydrate intake should be from complex carbohydrates found in vegetables, fruits, legumes, and whole grains. They contain fiber, vitamins, and minerals unlike simple carbohydrates that are devoid of nutrients; these are the carbohydrates you should avoid. Sugar, white bread, refined grains, chips, and fruit juices are all examples of simple carbs.

I can't afford healthy food. It's too expensive.

Take a step back for a moment and think about the big picture. Don't think in terms of your grocery bill alone. Remember that $117 billion that we spend on fast food? Let's also factor in the billions of dollars spent on obesity related health-care and prescription medications. When we change the way, we think about food, spending money on good food becomes an investment in our health. Most of us can afford real food if we take the time to reallocate our funds. Your well-being is worth it!

Staple plant-based foods like dried beans and rice is far less expensive than meat and poultry. Buy fruits and vegetables that are in season and on sale at your local super market. You don't have to shop at an expensive health food store.

Consider planting a garden and supplementing your cooking with your very own home-grown fruits and veggies. Create your own farm-to-table kitchen!

Multiple Seasons

I am so very proud of all of my patients and my team for their hard work, energy, dedication, passion, and commitment during the filming our documentary involving experiences related to a plant based diet in MS. Please take a moment to view our trailer. It can be found at: https://vimeo.com/311935402.

Helpful Hints:

❖ When you improve your general health, your neurological health will also improve.

❖ Maintaining a healthy weight is essential for MS patients.

❖ The standard American diet has a variety of health consequence like obesity, heart disease, high blood pressure, and diabetes. There is increasing evidence to suggest that saturated fats, omega-6 fatty acids, refined sugar, refined grains, and salt affect our immune system as well.

❖ The healthy bacteria in our gastrointestinal system is necessary for proper immune function.

❖ The foods we consume can alter the type of bacteria that is found in our intestines.

❖ Excess body fat secretes pro-inflammatory hormones.

❖ We recommend a whole-food, plant based diet.

Foods to Increase

- ➤ Vegetables
- ➤ Fruits
- ➤ Unrefined Whole Grains
- ➤ Beans
- ➤ Peas
- ➤ Lentils
- ➤ Nuts
- ➤ Seeds
- ➤ Leafy Greens

Foods to Avoid

- ➤ Meat
- ➤ Poultry
- ➤ Fish
- ➤ Refined Grains
- ➤ Eggs
- ➤ Refined Sugar
- ➤ Dairy
- ➤ Oils
- ➤ Convenience Food

10

EXERCISE

Exercise is another essential component of a healthy lifestyle, and its importance cannot be over stated. This holds true for everyone not just those with MS. Exercise decreases the risk of heart disease, high blood pressure, diabetes, osteoporosis, and a variety of other conditions.[132] For MS patients, exercise is essential to maintain and improve physical function and preserve independence. Physical deconditioning and muscle weakness can occur early in the disease course, and thus, timely intervention is key.[133] Exercise is not a mere recommendation; it is a medical intervention and needs to be viewed as such.[134]

Sedentary behavior has become our cultural norm, and it is a difficult cycle to break. We lead increasingly busy lives with very little down time, so it is often difficult to integrate new activities into our already crowded schedules. However, physical activity should be incorporated into our routine every single day to some degree. Many people have a negative association with the term exercise; they envision long hours at the local gym trying to use equipment alongside seasoned athletes. However, it is in fact a far broader term and encompasses a variety of activities.

Self-directed exercise routines, in which you choose your own workouts, are appropriate for most patients.[133] It is important to select a form of exercise that is accessible and enjoyable for you. As with dietary changes, the goal is long-term transformation, so start with small, realistic goals. Endurance training and resistance exercises have both been shown to provide benefit to MS patients.[135] Intuitively, an optimal exercise regimen includes a combination of cardio and resistance training, however, there is little data related to combined training in MS patients.[134]

For some, clinically supervised physical activity may be recommended by healthcare providers in an effort to tailor an exercise regimen to patients' individual physical capabilities and limitations.[134] This typically occurs in the form of formal physical therapy. Those who have ambulatory difficulties or require the use of a wheel chair do have unique challenges when it comes to exercise. However, regardless of your present physical abilities, there are ways to participate in physical activity safely.

Multiple sclerosis can make exercise more challenging due to fatigue, heat intolerance, and limited mobility. These are not reasons to avoid physical activity, but special considerations should be made.[134] For example, exercise can be broken down into short sessions if you are unable to tolerate large quantities at once. Start with 5-10 minute intervals followed by several minutes of rest. It is appropriate to exert yourself when exercising, but there can be a delicate balance between pushing yourself and overdoing it. One day of overly vigorous exercise may leave you nonfunctional the next day or two. For most, this boundary is not easily identifiable. It will likely take time and trial and error to find your own happy medium.

In the long run, exercise is beneficial for fatigue, but it can take several weeks to notice improvement in your energy level, so don't be discouraged. Staying cool during exercise is important in order to prevent worsening of your MS symptoms while you are working-out. As your core body temperature rises during exercise, some of your symptoms may become more prominent. This is not harmful and the increased symptoms will subside as your body cools back down with rest.[134] A variety of cooling strategies exist including drinking ice water before and during exercise, exercising indoors or during the cool morning hours, using cooling towels and personal fans, and wearing moisture wicking clothes.

We recommend an aerobic predominant exercise routine that incorporates low intensity weight training several days a week along with daily stretching. Aim for 30-60 minutes of activity at least 5 days a week. If this seems unrealistic for you, strive for 3 days a week initially.

Cardiovascular/Aerobic training

Cardiovascular training is any exercise that increases one's heart rate. It is generally broken down into high, moderate, and low intensity activities. These categories are based on how strenuous the activity is and how much physical effort is required.

High intensity

- ° Interval training: Run as fast as you can for 15- 30 seconds, jog for 2 minutes at a moderate paced. Repeat 3-5 times, resting for 5 minutes between each cycle.
- ° Circuit training: pick 5 exercises (push-ups, squats, lunges, dips, curls, mountain climbers, burpees, etc.), do as many as you can of one exercise for 20-30 seconds. Rest for 10 seconds then move on to the next exercise. Complete 3-5 cycles with 1 minute of rest in between each cycle.
- ° Go to a track: Run the straight edges and walk the curves. Aim for 4-8 laps
- ° Spin class, boxing class

Moderate intensity

- ° Jog a mile
- ° Jog for 30 seconds then walk for 2 minutes
- ° Repeat 5 times. Slowly increase your jogging interval to 1 minute
- ° Swimming laps at a comfortable pace
- ° Zumba or water aerobics
- ° Playing a game of tennis or pickup basketball

Low intensity

- ° Walking around the neighborhood
- ° Yoga, Tai Chi
- ° Leisurely bike ride
- ° Equine therapy
- ° Hiking
- ° Rock climbing

Weight/Resistance Training

Weight training is exercise completed against varying degrees of resistance with the goal of increasing strength and muscle mass. It also helps reduce fat by increasing your baseline metabolic rate and improves bone strength.[136, 137] For MS patients, there are specific muscle groups that should be targeted due to the nature of the disease. Damage caused from MS leads to weakness of the extensor muscles in the arms and the flexor muscles in the legs.[138, 139] Knowing this, can help make your time spent exercising more constructive. This doesn't mean that you should disregard other muscle groups all together, however, special attention should be given to these areas.

Proper form is important when you are learning any new exercise. Improper technique can lead to a variety of injuries. Before attempting a new weight lifting exercise, find a video on the proper form or consider booking time with a personal trainer to teach you appropriate technique. Initially, you may consider supervised weight training with a physical therapist or trainer to help ensure proper form and prevent injury.[134] Start with body weight exercises that rely on gravity to create resistance then work your way up to using weights or resistance bands. Begin with lighter weights that you can lift comfortably for 12-15 repetitions. If you are unable to maintain correct form, decrease the weight. Consider keeping an exercise journal to help track your progress. Write down which exercises you complete and the amount of weight used for each exercise. This will help ensure that you are not overworking certain muscle groups and can help guide you as you look to increase resistance.

Body Weight Strength Training Exercises: 3 sets of 10-15 repetitions each

- Squats
- lunges
- push-ups
- triceps
- dip
- pull-ups
- box jumps

Core strengthening exercises: 3 sets of 10-15 repetitions each.

- Sit ups
- Planks
- Bicycle crunch
- Mountain climbers
- Plank jacks
- Russian twist
- Reverse crunch
- Spider man plank

Extensors Muscles of the Arms

- ° Triceps
- ° Triceps kickbacks
- ° Triceps extensions
- ° Triceps pushups
- ° Lateral raise
- ° Front raise
- ° Plank row

Wrist Extensors

- Wrist extensions with a 2-3 pound weight or resistance bands

Finger Extensors

- Finger extensions using a resistance band

Flexor Muscles of the Legs

Hip Flexors

- Squats
- Sumo squats
- Sit-to-stands
- Step up
- Lunges
- Marching in place (try adding ankle weights)
- Wall sits
- Jump squat
- Tuck jumps

Knee Flexors

- Leg curls
- Dead lift
- Bridge/hip raise
- Plank with leg lift
- Lunges

- Donkey kicks

Dorsi-Flexor

- Foot extensions with a resistance band or kettle bell

It may take weeks to months to notice any tangible benefits from your exercise regimen, so do not become discouraged if you do not see immediate results. In time, routine physical activity is shown to improve strength, endurance, balance, fatigue, pain, depression, and cognitive function.[133, 140]

The importance of stretching can often be overlooked, and it should be viewed as more than a mere adjunct to routine exercise. Stretching can help improve flexibility, range of motion, and decrease the risk of injury.[141] It is particularly important for MS patients because they tend to have increased muscle tightness. One of the great things about stretching is that it can be done throughout the day at any time in any place.

When stretching, focus on major muscle groups and those that feel the tightest. It is important to hold each stretch for at least a minute a piece before moving on to the next muscle group.[141] While stretching properly is time consuming, it must be done on a consistent basis to be effective.

If exercise is new to you, there is a lot of information to take in, so we will highlight some general considerations as well. Ensure you have the proper equipment before starting your exercise routine. Supportive shoes are particularly important especially if you plan to do a fair amount of walking or jogging. Alternate the main focus of your workout; focus on legs one day, arms the next, and then your core. This will help add variety to your routine and will help keep you from overworking a single muscle group. Most importantly, stay positive! Working towards physical fitness takes time and determination.

Helpful Hints:

- ❖ Exercise does not have to mean going to the gym for an hour. The goal is to increase physical activity. It can be taking your dogs on a long walk or playing soccer with your kids at the park.

❖ Aim for 30-60 minutes of physical activity 5 days a week.

❖ Depending on your current activity level or degree of heat sensitivity, exercising for 30-60 minutes at one time may not be possible. It is reasonable to break up your exercise into smaller segments with periods of rest in between.

❖ Start easy-don't work out so hard that you become too sore and are less motivated to work out again the following day. Alternatively, being a little sore is a good thing! It shows that you are building muscle and making progress.

❖ Give yourself rest in between workouts to aid recovery.

❖ Stay hydrated. Drink water before, during, and after your workout.

❖ Staying cool during exercise is paramount. Drink ice water before you start working out to help lower your core body temperature from the beginning. Consider using a cooling towel or a personal fan while you exercise.

❖ Walk around the grocery store or mall if it is too warm to be outside.

❖ Many insurance plans offer gym memberships at reduced rates. Check with your insurance carrier before joining a gym.

❖ If you are on a tight budget, there are many free or low cost apps available that offer a variety of exercise recommendations. Check out YouTube videos, and many local libraries have exercise DVDs available for checkout. Workout in your garage, backyard, or a nearby park.

❖ There are a variety of community programs available for MS patients. Check with the National MS Society to see what is available in your area.

❖ Find a community of people to work out with as a group. This will help keep you accountable and will make exercise more enjoyable.

❖ It takes effort to become and stay motivated when it comes to being physically fit. Put motivational quotes on your mirror or save them as your phone background to help keep you inspired. Have a friend or family member send you encouraging text messages. Remember, even professional athletes have to motivate themselves to work out!

❖ If your fatigue is exceptionally bad on a given day, modify your workout to be lighter, but still do it! You will have more energy afterwards even though it may seem counterintuitive.

❖ Try listening to music while you exercise. Create a special playlist of your favorite upbeat songs to make the time pass more quickly.

❖ Yoga, pilates, and tai chi are excellent for those looking to improve balance. Modifications can be made for people at any level, so there is no excuse not to try it!

How do I know which exercises to do?

Ask your provider if they have any specific recommendations for you. Are there exercises you should avoid or focus on more? Start with those and expand from there.

How many repetitions of each exercise should I do?

This answer will vary from person to person. Aim for 2-3 sets of 10-15 reps knowing that you may not be able to complete this many. Ideally, you should complete as many reps as it takes to obtain a slight fatigue. When you reach that point, take a break and then try another set. You want to challenge yourself so you can improve, but you do not want to work so hard that you are completely exhausted. Remember the happy medium that we discussed previously. Experiment with different variations of sets, reps, and weight until you find something that is the perfect balance for you.

My MS symptoms seem to worsen while I exercise. Should I still continue to exercise?

Yes! As we discussed before, you may experience temporary worsening of your MS symptoms while exercising. This is not harmful, and the increased symptoms will subside as your body cools back down with rest.

Do I need to tell my fitness instructor/ personal trainer I have MS?

It is always up to you who you do and don't disclose your diagnosis to, however, in this instance it is likely to your advantage to divulge this information. Your trainer can better tailor your workout to your specific needs and better ensure your safety when they know your strengths and challenges.

I have weakness in one arm/leg. Should I only work out my weak side?

No, while you want to strengthen your weaker muscles, you also want to maintain the strength you have in other muscle groups. The number of reps performed should be increased at weaker muscle groups. This will allow for the weaker side to 'catch up' to the stronger side, reducing the overall magnitude of strength difference between muscle groups. The extent of exercise differences will differ from patient to patient. Be sure to discuss this with your personal trainer, healthcare team, physical therapist, etc.

11

OTHER LIFESTYLE MODIFICATIONS

When it comes to maintaining a healthy lifestyle, both diet and exercise are key. However, there are additional considerations to be made regarding non-MS specific interventions and lifestyle choices that optimize general health.

Smoking

It is well known that smoking cigarettes causes harm; there are a variety of toxic chemicals found in cigarette smoke including nicotine and nitric oxide and numerous other compounds. The long-term consequences of smoking are vast including cancer, emphysema, periodontal and heart disease.[142] While there is not a clear causal relationship between MS and tobacco use, associations have been made between smoking and MS disease course.[143, 144] Smoking may also affect one's response to disease modifying therapies and other symptomatic medications although this has not yet been formally studied.

Nicotine is highly addictive and can quickly become a means of self-medication.[142] For most, it is an enjoyable, social experience and a way manage with stress. Thus, it becomes both physically and emotionally addicting. Quitting smoking is one of the most difficult tasks anyone can accomplish. This is intensified by the fact that individuals experience both physical nicotine withdraw and the emotional withdraw of giving up a habit that has been a source of pleasure. While extremely difficult, quitting smoking can have both immediate and long term benefits. Smoking cessation now involves more than just nicotine gum or patches. It can include a multidisciplinary approach that incorporates health educators, social workers, and psychologists. Technology has also been leveraged with the use of mobile applications.[145, 146] If you are a current smoker, please consider speaking to your healthcare provider about quitting.

Managing stress

Life is inherently stressful. Between family commitments, professional responsibilities, and social obligations, we are constantly pulled in a dozen different directions, and stress can lead to physiological changes within the body. Having a chronic disease adds additional stress amongst appointments, medication management, physical/occupational/speech therapy, and daily symptoms. There is a myriad of tasks to tackle. For those with MS, they often experience amplified symptoms during periods of increased physical or emotional stress.

It is impossible to eliminate stress from our daily lives; there is simply no way around it. However, we can work to minimize angst. The first step is identifying what causes stress for you and isolating the sources of these stressors. Come up with a plan to address your concerns with each item, and embrace ways in which you can affect change. In circumstances where you cannot adjust the amount of stress, you can control your response to it. The way that you handle stress has the potential to encourage less healthy behavior, such as smoking, drinking too much alcohol, and overeating. It is important to identify and replace unhealthy coping strategies for healthy ones. There are a variety of strategies to employ. Formal counseling and mindfulness based interventions may be useful tools to help teach you additional stress management tactics.[147] Just like we have to train our bodies to be physically healthy, we have to train ourselves to be emotionally healthy.

Helpful Hints:

❖ Talk with someone about your anxieties whether it is a counselor, a trusted friend, or family member.

❖ Reflect on ways in which you can embrace more support into your life. Be present, invest in relationships, find ways to facilitate engagement, and allow others to help you navigate life's difficulties.

❖ Exercise is one of the best ways to help manage stress by releasing tension and frustration. Go on a long walk, get your heart rate up, and move!

❖ Allow yourself to have feelings. In our culture, we are conditioned to give others the perception that we are perpetually "fine". If we are honest with ourselves, we are rarely fine. We are almost always experiencing some emotion, which is entirely normal and healthy. Start by working towards identifying those feelings. Once that has become easier for you, try relaying them to a close friend.

❖ Use breathing techniques to help you relax and become more mindful. There are a variety of formal breath-based meditation methods that you can research online.

❖ Make yourself a priority. Set aside time for yourself and find things that you enjoy. Invest in a new hobby, read a book, or learn to play an instrument.

❖ Create goals. We often advise patients that achieving them is not always the intent for this recommendation. It involves the process, teachings throughout the journey and, more importantly, how we respond to failures if we fall short of them. This approach makes us better fighters for the future.

12

COMMON SYMPTOMS

The symptomatic presentation of MS can be highly variable from patient to patient depending on where lesions have occurred within the brain and spinal cord. Similarly, symptoms can be erratic and evolve over time. For patients, this often times produces additional frustration. Some symptomatic complaints can correlate to a specific lesion while other symptoms tend to be more global in nature and are likely not related to a single lesion. While symptoms will vary depending on the individual, they are typically well managed with medication and life style modifications.

Fatigue

Fatigue is one of the most common and often debilitating symptoms reported by MS patients. It affects nearly all MS patients at one time or another, yet we still do not fully understand the exact mechanism behind MS fatigue because it is multidimensional. Fatigue can be directly related to the disease process itself, which is known as primary MS fatigue, or a result of secondary causes like poor sleep, pain, medication side effects, and mood. This is known as secondary fatigue.[148-150]

Fatigue can be exceptionally hard to describe, and often patients tell me that 'you just know it when you feel it'. MS fatigue can have physical, mental, and psychological effects. Physical fatigue is the overwhelming sense of exhaustion that is unrelated to the amount of sleep one has had and is often independent of one's activity level. Mental fatigue can involve difficulty processing information, focusing, completing tasks, or organizing thoughts. Finally, emotional or psychological fatigue can inhibit one's ability to engage in activities and relationships or pursue hobbies or other interests.

Fatigue can be especially challenging for patients because it is pervasive and interferes with every aspect of life by limiting daily activities and social engagement. It is also invisible to everyone else, which can make it difficult for patients to get the support they need from friends and family.
In an effort to manage fatigue, it is imperative to make sleep a priority;

give yourself permission to rest. Energy conservation is also key, and you will need to learn to "budget" your energy well. You must prioritize what is most important to you and pace your activities throughout the day and throughout the week accordingly. Focus your energy on the things that are most important to you and your family first. Additionally, you may be able to identify specific tasks or activities that can be modified and completed in a more efficient manner.[149] Exercise can also help reduce fatigue over time, however, starting an exercise routine can be exceptionally difficult when you feel physically and mentally exhausted.[151] There are also medications such as modafinil, amantadine, stimulants, and supplements that your provider may recommend.[150, 152] There are special considerations that must be made prior to starting medication for fatigue (i.e. sleep disturbance, high blood pressure, underlying cardiac disease, etc.), and medication for fatigue is not appropriate for everyone. Using at least 3 different agents, and alternating between them during the week, helps keep your body from becoming tolerant to a single medication. Use a combination of prescribed medications, over the counter remedies, and caffeine. Keep in mind that not all agents will be equally effective in treating your fatigue.

Therefore, reserve the more effective ones for your extra busy days.

Ultimately, treatment should involve a multidisciplinary approach that incorporates exercise, energy conservation techniques, dietary changes, and self-care strategies.[150, 151, 153]

For additional information and tools pertaining to the surveillance and management of fatigue, be sure to refer to our other resource. (search MS Fatigue Fix in the App Store or Google Play)

Helpful Hints:

- ❖ Budget your energy wisely.

- ❖ Make time for yourself.

- ❖ Prioritize the activities you enjoy most.

❖ If your provider finds that medication is appropriate for your fatigue, consider alternating between several different medications. This ensures that your body does not develop a tolerance to a single agent.

❖ Rest when you need to and don't feel guilty about it!

❖ You will likely need to incorporate several different strategies to manage your fatigue.

Sleep Disorders

Sleep disturbance is another frequently reported problem amongst individuals with MS and is seen more frequently in MS patients when compared to the general population. Sleep disorders can also compound fatigue complaints.[154-156] Sleep disorders encompass a wide range of syndromes including insomnia, daytime sleepiness, periodic leg movements (PLM), restless legs syndrome (RLS), abnormal sleep–wake cycle, and breathing disorders, which have all been reported in MS patients.[156, 157] While poor quality of sleep may be related to a specific sleep disorder, a variety of factors can contribute to poor sleep quality.[157]

Insomnia is one of the more well-known disorders among the general population and can refer to difficulty initiating or maintaining sleep.[156] The most common complaint among patients is difficulty falling asleep, which can be attributed to a variety of causes like RLS, pain, depression, and anxiety.[155, 157] It may also be related to medication side effects or caffeine consumption. RLS and PLM occur more often in those with MS and can affect the time it takes one to fall asleep as well as duration of sleep.[158] Similarly, we know that those with depression and pain are more likely to experience poor sleep.[155]

Obstructive sleep apnea (OSA) is a common sleep disorder in which breathing frequently stops and restarts throughout the night.[159] While it is prevalent within the general population, it has been suggested that MS patients are more prone to OSA.[160] It is more likely to occur in those who are overweight, have a large neck, or have a small airway. If someone has mentioned that you snore, hold your breath, or gasp for air in your sleep, these are important signs to report to your provider because OSA tends to be under recognized in MS patients. This may be related to the level of fatigue that MS patients generally experience at baseline.[160] While there is not a direct cause and effect relationship established between MS and sleep breathing disorders, it is highly prevalent.[156, 160] It may be appropriate to refer you to a sleep specialist for a formal evaluation.

As previously mentioned, there are a variety of secondary causes that lead to sleep disruptions. For example, many patients wakeup frequently due to pain or get up to use the restroom. Simply being less active[161] or napping during the day can also lead to sleep disturbances. Medications are often a contributing factor as well; many commonly used prescriptions are known to be 'activating'.[156] Regardless of the cause, poor quality sleep can lead to excessive daytime sleepiness, which can further intensify preexisting fatigue. When we are chronically tired, we are not able to function our best physically or mentally. High quality sleep is necessary for physical and psychological restoration and must be a priority for those with MS.

Helpful Hints:

❖ Aim for at least 7-8 hours of sleep each night.

❖ Anxiety and depression are a frequent cause of insomnia. If you are waking in the night or having difficulty falling asleep without an identifiable cause, talk to your provider about your mood.

❖ Exercise! It encourages good sleep. However, do not exercise right before bedtime. The endorphins your body releases during exercise act like a stimulant and may make it difficult to sleep.

❖ Establish a routine. Go to bed and wake up at the same time every day. Your body is trainable over time.

❖ Do not drink caffeine after 2PM. The half-life of caffeine is 5 hours, so you need to allow time for it to get out of your system.[162]

❖ Stretch before getting into bed to help relax your muscles and your mind.

❖ Don't watch TV or use electronic devices in bed. These are stimulating and will keep you up. Associate your bed with sleep.

❖ Don't lay in bed for more than 20 minutes. If you are unable to fall asleep during that time, get up and go read quietly in another room.

❖ Consider keeping a sleep diary for a week or two to help identify and better understand what is interfering with your sleep.

Pain

MS patients can have a variety of pain complaints some of which are the result of MS and others that are not. Approximately half of patients report pain at one time or another. Differentiating between the two and isolating the cause can be challenging at times but important nonetheless.[163] Pain can range from mild to severe and can be perceived in a variety of ways. Common descriptors include sharp, stabbing, burning, aching, throbbing, electrical, squeezing, "pins and needles," and general discomfort. The character or type of pain can help to identify the cause.

Pain may be brief and only experienced for a few weeks to months, or it may be an enduring concern. There are a variety of medications available to treat nerve pain. Anticonvulsant (seizure) medications, mood medications, and anti-inflammatory agents are very helpful and tend to be less sedating than pure analgesic medications.[164] The use of opioid medications is typically reserved for refractory pain due to the addictive nature and possible side effects related to treatment. See below for further details regarding management of specific types of pain.

Paroxysmal symptoms

Paroxysmal symptoms are characterized by brief, frequent episodes where symptoms occur suddenly, often unexpectedly. While the symptoms are transient, they can appear repeatedly throughout the day. It is often described as an "electrical storm" because symptoms are the result of misfiring nerves. Symptoms that are paroxysmal in nature tend to occur for a period of weeks to months followed by a period of symptom inactivity, and symptoms recur periodically.[165]

Lhermitte's - is a common paroxysmal symptom that is the direct result of previous damage to the cervical spinal cord. It is an electrical sensation that starts at the base of the skull and radiates down the spine. Patients often describe it as a jolt of electricity running down their neck and back. Lhermitte's is triggered by bending the neck down toward the chest. The mechanical manipulation of the spinal cord that occurs when moving the neck forward causes misfiring of nerves in areas where there is scaring of the spinal cord. Symptoms are typically self-limited but can be treated with anticonvulsants (seizure medication).[164, 166]

Trigeminal neuralgia - is another common paroxysmal symptom that is described as a stabbing, ice pick like pain that occurs along the side of the face due to damage to the trigeminal nerve. Pain typically starts near the ear and travels down towards the jaw. It is exquisitely painful and can be quite distressing for those who suffer from it. Trigeminal neuralgia is often misinterpreted as dental pain and thus, it is important to differentiate the two. It can be treated with anti-convulsant (seizure) medications such as carbamazepine or oxcarbazepine. There are also surgical procedures available for cases that are refractory to medication.[164, 167]

Tonic spasms - are brief muscle contractions in the arms or legs that last for several seconds at a time. They can occur anywhere from a handful of times each day to a couple of hundred times throughout the day depending on the patient. While tonic spasms can be spontaneous, they are often triggered by sudden movement of the affected limb.[164] The anticonvulsant carbamazepine is the treatment of choice, and patients respond exceptionally well.[168] The medication can be stopped after 6-8 weeks if symptoms resolve and can be restarted in the future if symptoms recur.

Helpful Hints:

❖ Due to potential side effects of anticonvulsant (seizure) medications, always take your medication as it was prescribed by your provider.

❖ Never increase your medication on your own.

❖ Consult your provider if you feel that your current dose is inadequate.

❖ When you are instructed to increase a medication by your provider, it is best to stop at the lowest effective dose that controls your pain.

❖ You may be asked to repeat lab work until you are stable on your maintenance dose.

Spasticity

Spasticity is the feeling of tightness in the arms or legs that is caused by increased muscle tone. This is the result of inappropriate signally between the brain or spinal cord and the muscles. There is a loss of the inhibitory signal that tells the muscles to stop flexing or contracting. Spasticity is common for MS patients and can impact one's quality of life by producing pain or limiting mobility.[169] Over 80% of MS patients have encountered spasticity. Patients tend to find that fatigue, emotional stress, and cold temperatures make their spasticity worse. Understanding your own spasticity triggers can help improve management.[170]

Spasticity is best treated with a combination of medication and stretching/exercise.[169] Massage therapy may also be helpful.[171] Unfortunately, many of the medications used to treat spasticity are quite sedating. In time, patients tend to become tolerant of the side effects. For those who are unable to obtain relief with oral therapies, treatment with botulinum toxin injections and implantable baclofen pumps can be considered.[164, 172, 173]

Helpful Hints:

❖ Stretch every morning when you wake up and every evening before bed focusing on the muscle groups where you have the most discomfort.

❖ When stretching, hold each position for at least 1 minute before moving on to the next stretch.

❖ Urinary tract infections often make spasticity acutely worse. If you feel like your muscle spasm have worsened, contact your provider to help rule out an infection.

Weakness

Weakness may occur in any part of the body, but it is typically most prominent in the arms, legs, and core muscles. Weakness can be the direct result of damage to the brain and/or spinal cord, but it can also be the result of deconditioning due to inactivity and limited mobility.[174] Weakness that is the consequence of MS occurs because the brain is not able to effectively communicate with the corresponding muscles. Damage to the nervous system interferes with the signal between the brain and muscles. As mentioned in chapter eight, the specific muscles are directly affected. This includes the extensor muscles in the upper extremities (triceps, wrist extensors, and finger extensors) and the flexor muscles in the lower extremities (hip flexor, knee flexor, and dorsiflexor of the foot).[138, 139] Exercise training should be targeted to these muscle groups to help maintain strength and function.

Weakness due to inactivity, on the other hand, is not limited to these specific muscles; it can affect any muscle group. For general deconditioning, weight training and cardio is important to increase strength and stamina. Weakness, regardless of the cause, will interfere with daily function and ambulatory abilities, so it is important to address any reduction in strength sooner rather than later.[174] The longer you wait, the harder it is to regain function.

Helpful Hints:

❖ Focus your strength training on specific muscles groups

❖ Physical therapy can be very helpful to teach you specific exercises to improve muscle strength

❖ There may be assistive devices to help improve your functionality with yourself! You are not going to gain all of your strength back in one day. Small gains are valuable.

❖ Don't push yourself too hard. As we discussed earlier, start small and slowly increase your activity level/resistance. You do not want to cause an injury, which could lead to more inactivity.

Gait dysfunction

Limited mobility is a concern for most MS patients whether it is something they are fearful of in the future or a reality they live with on a daily basis. Everyone wants to ambulate independently, and the thought of that being disrupted is alarming. Several factors can contribute to walking difficulties including muscle weakness, spasticity, balance difficulties, changes in sensation in the feet and legs, and deconditioning.[174, 175]

Ambulatory difficulties can manifest as reduced walking speed, changes in gait mechanics, or poor endurance.[176] Sometimes people may have a perfectly normal gait when they start walking but can develop walking problems with prolonged ambulation or standing due to fatigue and poor endurance.

Improving overall physical fitness can help improve walking abilities in MS patients.[174, 176] An evaluation with a physical therapist can help determine the cause of gait difficulties, and they can construct a tailored exercise regimen to improve aerobic capacity and muscle strength as well as teach patients how to walk safely. Therapist can also assist in training patients how to use assistive devices properly. Improper technique is common and can lead to further gait dysfunction.

Walking difficulties can occur early in the disease course.[176] Regardless of the cause, it is important to identify subtle changes and intervene early. In my experience, patients wait until they are having significant trouble before they discuss their ambulatory difficulties with their providers. Similarly, patients tend to wait too long to consider assistive devices like a cane or walker. Do not wait until you are stumbling or having falls to discuss your walking concerns. It only takes one fall to have a potentially serious injury. The sooner an intervention can be implemented, the better your chances are for success. Research is underway to utilize wearable technology to assess for subtle gait changes.

Helpful Hints:

❖ Consider physical therapy for gait or balance training.

❖ Often times, patients wait too long to incorporate assistive devices. The reality is that these devices allow you to ambulate safely and enhance independence.

❖ If you are having difficulty walking, it is important to continue walking as much as you can safely. If you do not use those muscles routinely, they will become increasingly more weak.

❖ If your gait dysfunction is related to spasticity, ensure that you are stretching routinely and that your spasticity is being managed appropriately.

❖ Ask your provider if Ampyra (a medication that improves walking) is appropriate for you.

❖ If you have foot drop, there are several adaptive devices that may be of assistance; these include ankle foot orthosis and e-stim devices like the Bioness.

Cognitive impairment

Many patients with MS will experience some degree of cognitive impairment at some point in their disease course; anywhere from 40-70% of individuals with MS report cognitive difficulties.[177-179] It is important to note that these changes can occur early in the disease and in the absence of physical disability.[177, 180] The brain has a variety of advanced functions that allow information to become meaningful to us. We tend to not recognize the complexity of these functions until something goes wrong. The brain is responsible for attention, memory, speech, language, processing, and decision making along with managing and synthesizing information. Knowing the eloquent functions involved, it makes sense that

MS lesions can interrupt these tasks. Specific cognitive challenges will vary amongst individuals depending on lesion location and lesion volume. However, there are certain functions that tend to be more affected than others. The ability to learn, long-term memory, multitasking, and focus one's attention are common deficiencies. Processing speed and abstract reasoning are also affected.[177, 179]

Aside from overall lesion burden, we also know that a variety of factors confound cognitive difficulties; fatigue, depression and medications are a few examples.[177, 179] Additionally, the brain atrophies at a faster rate in those with MS when compared to the general population.[181, 182] Changes in the brain's structure, whether from atrophy or from the lesions themselves, can alter cognitive function.[183]

Neuropsychological testing can be beneficial to help determine specific problem areas for those who have cognitive complaints. Baseline testing early in the disease course is beneficial, so that you can gauge change over time and timely intervention is key.[179] Sometimes there are interventions available to help with specific deficiencies identified, like treating fatigue or depression. Other times, coping strategies are recommended like reducing stress, making notes, setting cell phone reminders. Depending on where you live, you may have access to cognitive rehabilitation therapy, which is like physical therapy for your brain. A therapist can work with you to learn new strategies to compensate for changes in cognition. Employing novel approaches to improve focus and minimize confusion, can go a long way. Stress, fatigue, and mood changes will amplify thinking difficulties, so it is important to make sure these are adequately addressed. There are some prescription medications available for memory, however, their utility is highly variable depending on the patient.[177, 179]

Helpful Hints:

❖ Once cognitive changes have occurred, full recovery is unlikely. Patients must learn to compensate by making notes, using cell phone reminders, and employing other compensatory measures.

❖ Aerobic exercise has been shown to be valuable for cognitive function.

❖ If you are a student, consider requesting additional time for exams and standardized testing.

❖ Engaging in activities that make you think can help maintain cognitive function. Examples include doing crossword puzzles or playing Sudoku. Learning to play an instrument or speak a foreign language is also something to consider.

Vertigo

Dizziness is a common complaint for MS patients, and it is important to differentiate between lightheadedness and vertigo. Vertigo is the sensation that the room is spinning versus feeling faint and unsteady. Vertigo may be the result of a lesion in the brainstem or cerebellum. It may also be caused by disorders of the inner ear.

Dizziness, on the other hand, is more often the result of blood pressure fluctuations, heart rhythm abnormalities, low blood sugar, or medication side effects. It is important to rule other conditions out before attributing dizziness to MS.

Identifying the cause of vertigo and/or dizziness is the first step to employing the most appropriate treatment. There are several medications available to address vertigo, which will vary depending on the individual patient and provider.

Headaches

Many patients with MS suffer from headache events, including both migraine headaches and tension headaches though headaches are not generally considered a symptom of MS. Studies suggests that MS patients are not more prone to headaches when compared to the general population although this claim has been debated.[184, 185]

There are a variety of treatments available to address headaches and potentially prevent them from occurring. This is very individualized, so speak with your provider about managing your headaches. It is also important to note that headaches can be a side effect of you MS therapy.[186]

Helpful Hints:

❖ Make sure that you are getting plenty of rest. Lack of sleep with increase headache frequency.

❖ Drink plenty of water. Dehydration can cause headache events.

❖ Do not take over the counter medications like acetaminophen or ibuprofen every day. This can lead to rebound headaches.

❖ Stress is frequently a contributing factor. Recognizing and reducing stress may help reduce headache frequency.

❖ Certain supplements like magnesium and riboflavin may be helpful in preventing headaches.

Mood Changes

Emotional health tends to be neglected in our society as a whole. As a culture, we are highly focused on physical health but often do not address emotional well-being, which is equally as important. Mood disorders are common for MS patients and should be addressed when present as they contribute to overall quality of life. While there is an emotional component to being diagnosed with a chronic disease, there can be emotional consequences of the disease that extend beyond grieving the diagnosis.

Depression and anxiety are one of the most common challenges experienced by MS patients. These symptoms can be present even in individuals with mild MS, and some of the medications used to treat the disease are associated with depression.[187, 188] However, depression and anxiety are not always recognized clinically by physicians and other healthcare providers, and in my experience, patients tend to be hesitant to acknowledge mood related concerns as a result of social stigma.
Depression can have a variety of presentations that extend beyond just sadness. For some, it manifests as irritability, lack of motivation/interest, and changes in appetite.

Depression can also contribute to cognitive changes, pronounced fatigue, and sleep disturbance. Depression is not always easily identifiable and differentiating between depression and MS symptoms can be difficult. However, recognizing that there is a mood disturbance is crucial because there are many effective treatment options that can improve your quality of life.[187] There are a variety of medications that help by changing the chemical environment in the brain.

They work by increasing the chemical serotonin, dopamine, or norepinephrine, which are responsible for maintaining a balanced mood. Generally speaking, these medications are well tolerated and can have a profound impact for those with clinical depression. Counseling and cognitive behavioral therapy (CBT) may be recommended either independently or in combination with medication management.[188, 189] Working with a skilled psychotherapist, can help one recognize the source of their depression and work towards healing. Exercise has also been shown to improve depressive symptoms.[140]

Anxiety is characterized by undue levels of self- inflicted stress, worry, and fear of the future. Some degree of anxiety is normal, and it is our natural response to challenging life circumstances. However, persistent, overwhelming anxiety that interferes with daily activities can be debilitating. Like depression, it is common in MS patients, and it is often compounded by the uncertainty of living with an unpredictable disease. Physical manifestations of anxiety can include heart palpitations, shakiness, upset stomach, and difficulty sleeping. For MS patients, treating anxiety is particularly important. Heightened stress and anxiety can lead to medication non-compliance, and it can also amplify MS symptoms, which in turn further increases one's anxiety.[187]

Identifying anxiety is the first step to successful treatment. If you find yourself preoccupied with the outcome of future events, avoiding social situations, or being hyper focused on controlling your circumstances, you likely have some degree of anxiety. In my experience, treatment is most fruitful with the combination of medication management and the implementation of stress reduction techniques, which is best done with the assistance of a psychotherapist.[187, 188]

Euphoria, unlike depression, is characterized by excessive feelings of happiness that do not fit life's circumstances. This is exceedingly rare in

MS but does occur. Patients are unrealistically joyful and experience elation with everyday activities. There is not a specific treatment strategy for this disorder as it tends to be associated with cognitive impairment and poor insight.[190]

Pseudobulbar affect (PBA) is a rare neurological disorder where one experiences uncontrollable emotional outbursts. Individuals will have outbreaks of laughing or crying that are inappropriate for the given situation and do not mirror how they are actually feeling. The treatment for this disorder is highly specific and differs from that of depression and anxiety. While traditional mood medications may be considered, the medication dextromethorphan/quinidine is the first therapy specifically approved for treating PBA.[191-193]

Becoming emotionally healthy takes work. We often strive for our bodies to become physically healthy by adopting healthy diets and implementing exercise regimens, and we must employ similar effort to become emotionally healthy. It will not happen on its own.

Helpful Hints:

- ❖ Receiving treatment for depression or anxiety does not mean that you are weak.

- ❖ Some medications can increase emotional lability. Steroids, for instance, are notorious for this. Being aware of possible medication side effects, is important.

- ❖ Take time out of your day for meditation or thoughtful reflection.

- ❖ Limit caffeine intake if you are feeling anxious. It is a stimulant and can amplify anxiety and irritability.

- ❖ Exercise! As we have discussed previously, this is one of the best ways to manage stress.

- ❖ Recognize that you cannot control everything and perfection is unrealistic. Have realistic expectations for yourself.

❖ Starting medication for your depression or anxiety, does not mean that you are committed to it for the rest of your life. You may be able to discontinue it in the future.

Autonomic dysfunction

The autonomic system is part of the nervous system that is outside of voluntary control. It controls involuntary functions like temperature regulation, blood pressure control, heart rate, and bladder and bowel function. In MS patients, the autonomic nervous system can be damaged from demyelination and axonal loss in the brain or spinal cord. Treatment is aimed towards relief of symptomatic complaints, however, a formal autonomic evaluation may be recommended.[194]

Bladder Dysfunction

Bladder dysfunction is extremely prevalent within the MS patient population; most patients will be affected with bladder symptoms at one time or another. Patients may have issues with storing urine, emptying their bladder, or even a combination of the two. Storage difficulties are the result of an overactive bladder due to spasms within the bladder muscle. Urinary urgency and frequency are the manifestations of bladder spasms. Patients also complain of waking frequently during the night to use the bathroom (nocturia). Treatment should involve several tactics including medication management, physical therapy, timed voiding, and avoiding bladder irritants. On the other hand, urinary retention is characterized by the inability to empty the bladder completely or effectively. This is the result of sphincter muscles not being able to fully relax. Subsequently, the residual urine that does not get emptied is a breeding ground for bacteria and places patients at increased risk for urinary tract infections. If your provider suspects that this is an issue, they will likely recommend an ultrasound of your bladder to measure the volume of urine that remains in the bladder after being emptied. Certain medications may be helpful for improving bladder function. If bladder symptoms are not alleviated with first line treatments, a referral to urology is recommended for further evaluation and more sophisticated testing and alternate treatment options like botulism toxin injections.[194, 195]

Optimizing bladder function is especially important because it directly effects patients' independence, self-esteem, and quality of life. **Patients who have bladder dysfunction frequently endorse altering their social activities, work activities, and sleep patterns to accommodate for their bladder symptoms. Furthermore, they are at increased risk for other health conditions like urinary tract infections and skin break down. The good news is that treatment interventions are effective. Remember to be patient; it may take a little time to find an individualized treatment plan that works best for you.**

Helpful Hints:

❖ Be honest with your provider about your symptoms. They will be unable to help you if you are not entirely honest about what you are experiencing.

❖ Avoid bladder irritants; they can contribute to urinary urgency and frequency: caffeine, alcohol, acidic and spicy foods. You can find a more comprehensive list online.

❖ Limit fluids 3 hours prior to bedtime and void immediately prior to getting into bed

❖ Keep a change of clothes in your car or office in the event that you do have an accident

❖ Practice timed voiding. Go to the restroom every 2 hours whether you feel like you need to go or not.

❖ Make sure you are drinking at least 64 ounces of water a day.

Bowel Function

Bowel dysfunction is another common problem that can also greatly influence patients' quality of life. Bowel dysfunction is an overarching term that can encompass diarrhea, involuntary loss of stool, or constipation. A variety of factors can contribute to bowel function including decreased intestinal motility due to damage within the nervous system, structural abnormalities of the intestines, diet, fluid intake, physical immobility, and medications. Treatment is centered around medication management and biotherapy feedback.[196]

Helpful Hints:

❖ Make sure you are drinking at least 64 ounces of water each day. Being well hydrated is important to keep stools soft.

❖ Exercise! Physical activity promotes intestinal motility.

❖ Increase your dietary fiber; aim for 25-30 grams each day. This may require supplementing fruits and vegetable with a fiber powder.

❖ Discuss your medications with your provider.
❖ Many prescription medications can contribute to constipation.

❖ There are prescription and over the counter medications used to treat constipation that is refractory to the above tips. Check with your provider before you start any medication. Some are not safe to take long-term.

Sexual dysfunction

Sexual dysfunction is present upwards of 80% of MS patients, however, it is often underreported and subsequently undertreated despite being a major component of quality of life and self-esteem.[138, 197, 198] Sexual dysfunction may be the direct consequence of the disease itself, but is can also be caused by medication side effect, physical symptoms like fatigue, pain, and spasticity, or psychological factors. MS may directly damage the pathways responsible for sexual response, which can manifest as decreased arousal, difficulty achieving orgasm, or impaired lubrication.

Additionally, sensory deficits can lead to painful or impaired sensation, which can also limit sexual response.[197, 199, 200] Erectile and ejaculatory dysfunction are also commonly reported in men.[198] It is often difficult to identify the primary cause of sexual dysfunction because it tends to be multifactorial.[197, 199, 200] As always, it is important to remember that MS may not be the cause of every symptom. It may be worth having your hormone levels assessed by your primary care physician to rule out other medical causes. Major life changes like pregnancy or career changes can also contribute to decreased sexual desire.

There are medications available to treat erectile dysfunction and female sexual dysfunction. However, combination therapy incorporating medical interventions, sex therapy, education, and mood optimization typically works best and should involve a multidisciplinary approach.[197, 198]

Helpful Hints:

❖ Communicate openly with your partner; this fosters intimacy. Consider counseling or sex therapy if you need someone to help facilitate conversation.

❖ Exercise. It enhances mood and improves self-image.

❖ Limit alcohol intake.

❖ Use a lubricant to help reduce pain and dryness.

❖ Consider sexual stimulation techniques to enhance arousal.

❖ Certain medications, especially some antidepressants, can contribute to sexual dysfunction. Discuss possible medication side effects with your provider.

❖ For women, it may be beneficial to be evaluated by an urogynecologist who specializes in female sexual dysfunction.

Heat Sensitivity

It is VERY common for MS patients to be sensitive to environmental temperatures. Aside from finding the heat to be uncomfortable, many patients experience temporary worsening of their symptoms when exposed to the heat or humidity. Even small fluctuations can have a profound impact on patients' symptoms. Symptoms return to baseline once the aggravating source is removed and the body is able to cool back down. Cooling down can have quick and dramatic effects.[201] Uhthoff's phenomenon is a term used to describe this transient worsening of MS symptoms related to heat exposure. Basically, symptoms can increase with any activity that causes an elevation in core body temperature. This can occur due to warm weather outside, taking a warm shower, sitting in a hot tub, having a fever, or exercising. Some patients even notice worsening of their symptoms around the time of their menstrual cycle.[202] It is important to note that while most MS patients are heat sensitive, some patients have more difficulty with colder weather. These patients typically note increased spasticity and muscle pain. The take home message for all patients is to learn how your body responds to various environments and do your best to avoid extreme temperatures.

Helpful Hints:

❖ Stay indoors in the air conditioning during periods of extreme heat and humidity.

❖ Wear a cooling vest or other cooling products when you are out in the heat.

❖ Drink ice water or take a cool bath prior to going outdoors.

❖ Take an umbrella with you to create extra shade.

❖ Carry a personal fan and/or misting device.

❖ Park your car in the shade when possible and put a sun shade in your window shield.

❖ Keep a small ice chest will cool drinks in the car if you are going to be out running errands in the heat.

❖ Take a fever reducer when you are ill to help lower your core body temperature.

Everyone with MS has a unique experience, therefore, one's treatment journey will be equally unique. When it comes to managing MS related symptoms, it is important to remember that our medical treatments are not perfect and often times a multimodal approach incorporating diet, exercise, and other lifestyle modifications is essential for success.

13

FAMILY PLANNING

Many patients with MS are of childbearing potential and are looking to start or grow their families. There is a lot of misinformation regarding pregnancy and family planning for MS patients. There is no contraindication to pregnancy, and the reality is that MS patients tend to do really well during pregnancy.[203] Similarly, MS does not affect fertility for either men or women.[204] The biggest consideration when contemplating family planning is when to stop your disease modifying therapy and other symptomatic medications that could be harmful for the baby during pregnancy. Generally speaking, it is recommended that women stop their DMT for a couple of months prior to trying to conceive. However, this recommendation varies greatly among providers and is dependent upon one's current DMT, and the time off therapy should be minimized as much as possible.[205] Certain medications like teriflunomide (Aubagio) require special consideration and planning while glatiramer acetate (Copaxone) is generally considered safe to continue while trying to conceive.[206] It is important to discuss your plans for pregnancy with your provider before discontinuing your medication. For men, most medications are safe and are not harmful for the fetus. Teriflunomide is the exception and should be discontinued prior to conceiving.[39] Additionally, many symptomatic medications used to treat MS symptoms are not safe to continue during pregnancy.

Should you become pregnant while on MS therapy, there are pregnancy registries aimed at following the outcomes of these pregnancies. Registries for some medications are closed, and the results can be viewed online.

While the shift in hormones during pregnancy tends to provide protection from new disease activity during pregnancy, especially in the last trimester, it is possible to have a relapse during pregnancy.[203] In the event that new symptoms present themselves, contact your provider. It is safe to receive steroid treatment for a relapse while pregnant.

At the time of delivery, there are not any specific management strategies. Pregnant women with MS are not considered to have high risk pregnancies or deliveries. Anesthesia medications used for cesarean sections and pain management are equally safe for MS patients as the general population.[205] Some patients who have reduced muscle strength or impaired sensation, may have difficulty pushing during delivery.

Following delivery, patients are at an increased risk of developing new MS symptoms the first 3 months of the post-partum period.[203] Therefore, post-partum planning is key and best done at least a month prior to delivery. Many patients choose to breast-feed and, thus, remain off MS therapy. Our current MS therapies are not approved for use while breast feeding. Many neurologists recommend using Copaxone while breastfeeding, but this is not formally approved by the FDA. Therefore, other management strategies are employed for those who choose to breastfeed. Most patients choose to not to be exposed to a DMT during this time, but it is a very personalized decision.[207] However, it is generally recommended to receive either intravenous immunoglobulin (IVIG) or pulses of high dose steroids prophylactically for the first few months following delivery.[208, 209]

IVIG is a blood product consisting of pooled immune globulin from healthy individuals. The IVIG helps to regulate patient's over active immune system, and hopefully prevent relapses from occurring. The infusions are typically administered within one week of delivery and continued every 4-6 weeks while patients breastfeed. Insurance does not always approve IVIG, so it is recommended to start the approval process early. High dose steroids are a less expensive alternative to IVIG if insurance approval cannot be obtained. They are typically prescribed for three consecutive days once a month for the first few months following delivery. Dosing schedules will vary depending on the treating provider. It is recommended that patients receive their first dose within 1 week of delivery when possible.[208] IVIG and steroids are both safe to receive while breast-feeding, but check with your pediatrician for specific recommendations. As soon as patients are done breastfeeding, it is advised that they restart a disease modifying therapy.

Some old MS symptoms may be amplified during the post-partum period.

These symptoms may seem more intense due to the fatigue and stress of caring for a new baby. Therefore, it is important to prioritize your health as well and make time for rest.

The take home message is that having MS does not affect your ability to have a family. There are however considerations to be made, which take time to plan. If you are contemplating pregnancy, allow ample time and speak to your provider about devising a plan.

Helpful Hints:

- ❖ Pregnancy is safe, and MS patients tend to do well during pregnancy.

- ❖ Planning is key when it comes to pregnancy and MS.

- ❖ Different providers have different strategies for post-partum management. There is not a single "right" way of doing things.

- ❖ MRIs should be postponed until after delivery if possible.

- ❖ Should a MRI with contrast be needed while breastfeeding, it is recommended that patients pump and dump for a minimum of 24 hours following contrast exposure.

14

EXPERT ADVICE

Best Advice from Dr. Okuda:

Disease behavior related to multiple sclerosis has changed considerably as compared to 5, 10, and 15 years ago. Patients with MS are now experiencing less relapses, in general, for reasons that are unclear. Be optimistic. The diagnosis of MS may provide a wonderful opportunity to improve your general health and outlook on life.

The risk for new MS activity is highest in younger age groups. Starting on a FDA approved treatment as early as possible will give you the best chance for great outcomes.

The successful treatment of MS is not solely dependent on a single medication, diet, exercise philosophy, supplement, or mental outlook. Effectively addressing factors that significantly affect your well-being beyond any challenges that you may face as a patient with MS is key.

Focus on a set of goals. I encourage all patients to set goals for themselves whether it relates to understanding their condition, applying solutions for managing symptoms and energy reserves, or improving one's general health. At times setting multiple goals in different categories of life is beneficial. Not all of your goals may be accomplished, but this is not a problem as additional knowledge will be gained as you continue to challenge yourself.

In my opinion, refrain from continually seeking online information regarding your condition. Instead, focus on improving your life in some way. If you do find something that intrigues you online regarding new research or treatment intervention, ask your healthcare team about it during your next visit. Or, consider scheduling a visit for a longer, more in depth, discussion.

Be your own champion when it comes to your medical records. Although electronic medical record systems exist in nearly all health-care facilities, not all of them may be connected and when they are, finding relevant data for your care may be similar to piecing together a novel after searching through an unabridged dictionary. Having your own records of recent hospital stays, MRI studies on disk, prior clinic visits from other practitioners, and diagnostic study results will get you far.

Find a MS specialist who you feel you comfortable working with. Also, please keep in mind that your healthcare providers are people and patients too and some days at work are better than others. If you feel that a certain symptom or aspect of your care is not being fully addressed at the visit, please mention it. I always encourage all of my patients to be as forthcoming as possible so that we can arrive at a number of strategies to solve the problem

Best Advice from Katy:

You can do great things, and you are capable of more than you realize! MS does not own you! So, don't allow your diagnosis to define who you are. Be socially engaged, participating in activities that you enjoy helps you to see past your diagnosis and daily symptoms.

We have so many great MS therapies, but none of them are perfect. Effective treatment requires disease modifying therapies paired with a healthy diet and consistent exercise.

A positive attitude can significantly impact your experience!

Imagine that your daily MS symptoms are like the music playing out of your stereo. Your overall attitude and outlook can impact the "volume" of these symptoms on a daily basis. You have the power to decide whether they are going to be the primary focus of the day or just background noise.

Invest time in learning to manage your emotions. It is a skill that must be cultivated, and it does not happen overnight. Discouragement, fear, anxiety, and depression can all be expected at one time or another, but these feelings should not define who you are or your experience. Never be afraid to ask for help! There are so many services available for support.

I cannot over emphasize the importance of individual patient responsibility in the management of MS. You have the opportunity to play a key role in directing your care plan in partnership with your healthcare provider!

It is our responsibility to give you the knowledge, tools, and courage to take your health into your own hands. Invest in yourself!

Best Advice from Mandy:

Most nurses chose their profession because they wanted to help others. I know it may not always seem like it, but we are on your side. Nurses are most often the driving force behind the operation. They are the roles who implement what the providers have recommended. We are here to help you and sometimes that means setting boundaries and standards for your safety.

Please understand that there are multiple patients calling and sending electronic messages, and we have to help the patients with urgent issues first. We will get to your phone call or electronic message as soon as possible.

Therefore, when you call your providers office, please provide detailed and comprehensive information. It is helpful for the nurse when triaging phone calls. This will in turn help you, if you're having an urgent issue.

We are a team, and we want the best for you!

When it comes to needing a refill for one of your prescribed medications, it is recommended that you request a refill at least a week in advance. It can be stressful for both the patient and healthcare team if a patient waits until they are completely out of medication to request a refill.

Please keep in mind, that certain medications require routine lab monitoring, so you may be asked to have updated labs completed prior to receiving a refill. This is for your safety not to create frustration.

It is important to know what medications you are currently taking (the dosage and frequency) and why you are taking the medication. Please advise your healthcare team if you have questions or negative side effect from a medication. Do not stop taking the medication or change the dosage without consulting your healthcare team first. This is once again for your safety. Each medication has a maximum dosage that is deemed to be safe and exceeding that dose can be detrimental.

Because we are a team and you, as a patient, are a vital part of that team, we need to know if you do not agree with your treatment plan. We are relying on you to follow through with the plan just like you are relying on us to do the same. You will be more successful if you rake ownership of your healthcare.

You and your caregivers are the best advocates for your healthcare.

Your healthcare providers are a part of your support team, but they cannot be your only source of support.

We want you to have a support team around you to help manage your medications, transportation, emotional support, etc. You can build your support team with family, friends, neighbors, support groups, religious communities and more.

Physical exercise is important both for physical and mental health. Even going for a 5-10 minute walk outside can improve your mood and get you moving at the same time.

You have to make your health a priority. In order to be successful in caring for your family and friends, you have to take care of yourself.

15

RESOURCES

There are a multitude of resources available for those with multiple sclerosis. With the appropriate tools, MS can become just a small part of your life, allowing you to have a full, productive life. While this is not an exhaustive list, we have tried to make it as comprehensive as possible. Our field is ever evolving and with that comes the development of new patient support systems and programs, so always ask your provider or friends if they are aware of additional resources.

We recommend that you utilize well-known websites for both information regarding MS and available resources. Using group Facebook pages or blogs typically highlight experiences that are unique to individual patients.

Here is a list of organizations where you can find reliable information regarding MS.

The National Multiple Sclerosis Society, Multiple Sclerosis Association of America, and the MS Foundation
They have a variety of education material available about MS, symptoms, therapies, and local resources.

MS Coalition
This is a network of independent MS organizations that have joined together to create a central website for various resources offered to MS patients.

Can DO MS
Resources for emotional well-being, diet, and exercise.

Multiple Sclerosis Encouragement Organization
Provides inspiration and empowerment to people affected by MS and their care partners.

There are also number of organizations that provide caretaking services:

Home Watch Caregivers

Department of Aging and Disability Services (DADS)
You may apply for home aide services on their website.

Veteran Aide Services
Provides aide and attendant services for service connected veterans.

National Family Caregiver's Association
Resources for caregivers that include videos, checklists, and educational material.

National Caregiver's Library

Advocacy organizations are designed to help patients continue working and living a rewarding life. You can utilize these organizations to help with work accommodations:

Equal Employment Opportunity Commission

Job Accommodation Network (JAN) (Office of Disability Employment Policy of the US Department of Labor)

National Mobility Equipment Dealer's Association

Association for Driver Rehabilitation Specialists

As you may know there are always new disease modifying therapies being introduced to the market, so before long, this list will no longer be comprehensive. Each drug company has material concerning their products as well as information regarding their patient assistance programs online.

Here is a list of the current medications and their assistance program.

Genzyme: Aubagio and Lemtrada
MS One to One
Phone: 855-676-6326

Biogen: Avonex, Plegridy, Tecfidera, and Tysabri
MS Active Source

Phone: 800-456-2255

Bayer: Betaseron
Beta Plus
Phone: 800-788-1467

Teva: Copaxone
Shared Solutions
Phone: 800-887-8100

Novartis: Extavia
Extavia Go Program
Phone: 866-925-2333

Novartis: Gilenya
Gilenya Go Program
Phone: 877-408-4974

Sandoz: Glatopa
Glatopa Care
Phone: 855-452-8672

Genentech: Ocrevus
Genentech Access Program
Phone: 866-422-2377

EMD Serono: Rebif
MS Lifelines
Phone: 877-447-3243

Additional resources for medication assistance:

Mallinckrodt: AcTHar Gel
AcTHar Support and Access Program
Phone: 888-435-2284

Acorda Therapeutics: Ampyra
Ampyra Patient Support Services
Phone: 888-881-1918

Assistance programs for other prescription medications:

Good Rx
Phone: 888-277-3911

Needy Meds
Phone: 800-503-6897

Rx Hope

Teva Cares
Phone: 877-237-4881

Patient Access Network
Phone: 866-316-7263

Copay assistance programs for appointments and imaging:

Multiple Sclerosis Foundation
Provides a wealth of resources including financial assistance for office visits, free cooling vests or home care assistance. You can call 888-673-6287 or go to their website for additional information.

As you may know there are always new disease modifying therapies being introduced to the market, so before long, this list will no longer be comprehensive. Each drug company has material concerning their products as well as information regarding their patient assistance programs online. Here is a list of the current medications and their assistance program.

Multiple Sclerosis Association of America (MSAA) offers financial assistance for those how are unable to afford routine imaging. They also provide general information and resources. They can be reached online or by calling 800-532-7667.

There are a variety of cooling devices for those who are heat sensitive. This is by no means an exhaustive list but a good place to start investigating which devices would be most helpful for you:

MS Foundation (Cooling Program)
Coolture
Phone: 716-575-7294

Polar Products
Phone: 800-763-8423

Steele
Phone: 888-783-3538

These organizations empower patients to be physically active and meet their exercise goals:

Neurofitness Foundation
Phone: 817- 571-1323

Move Forward

We've discussed the importance of stress reduction, and here are a few tools to help you cope and manage anxiety:

www.calm.com

www.healthjourneys.com

www.drmiller.com

I'm Fine: A Real Feelings Journal by Dianne Jones

REFERENCES

1. Compston A, Coles A. Multiple sclerosis. Lancet 2008;372:1502-1517.

2. Keegan BM, Noseworthy JH. Multiple sclerosis. Annu Rev Med 2002;53:285-302.

3. Munger KL, Levin LI, Hollis BW, Howard NS, Ascherio A. Serum 25-hydroxyvitamin D levels and risk of multiple sclerosis. JAMA 2006;296:2832-2838.

4. Levin LI, Munger KL, O'Reilly EJ, Falk KI, Ascherio A. Primary infection with the Epstein- Barr virus and risk of multiple sclerosis. Ann Neurol 2010;67:824-830.

5. Marrie RA. Environmental risk factors in multiple sclerosis aetiology. Lancet Neurol 2004;3:709-718.

6. Pietrangelo A HV. Multiple Sclerosis by the numbers: facts, statistics, and you [online]. Available at: http://www.healthline.com/health/multiple-sclerosis/facts-statistics-infographic. Accessed 05/31/ 2017.

7. Weinshenker BG. Epidemiology of multiple sclerosis. Neurol Clin 1996;14:291-308.

8. Ross AP, Ben-Zacharia A, Harris C, Smrtka J. Multiple sclerosis, relapses, and the mechanism of action of adrenocorticotropic hormone. Front Neurol 2013;4:21.

9. Dyment DA, Ebers GC, Sadovnick AD. Genetics of multiple sclerosis. Lancet Neurol 2004;3:104-110.

10. Polman CH, Reingold SC, Banwell B, et al. Diagnostic criteria for multiple sclerosis: 2010 revisions to the McDonald criteria. Annals of neurology 2011;69:292-302.

11. Garg N, Smith TW. An update on immunopathogenesis, diagnosis, and treatment of multiple sclerosis. Brain Behav 2015;5:e00362.

12. Trapp BD, Peterson J, Ransohoff RM, Rudick R, Mork S, Bo L. Axonal transection in the lesions of multiple sclerosis. The New England journal of medicine 1998;338:278-285.

13. Confavreux C, Vukusic S. Natural history of multiple sclerosis: a unifying concept. Brain 2006;129:606-616.

14. Okuda DT, Srinivasan R, Oksenberg JR, et al. Genotype-Phenotype correlations in multiple sclerosis: HLA genes influence disease severity inferred by 1HMR spectroscopy and MRI measures. Brain : a journal of neurology 2009;132:250-259.

15. Thompson AJ, Banwell BL, Barkhof F, et al. Diagnosis of multiple sclerosis: 2017 revisions of the McDonald criteria. The Lancet Neurology 2017.

16. Polman CH, Reingold SC, Edan G, et al. Diagnostic criteria for multiple sclerosis: 2005 revisions to the "McDonald Criteria". Ann Neurol 2005;58:840-846.

17. Lublin FD, Reingold SC. Defining the clinical course of multiple sclerosis: results of an international survey. National Multiple Sclerosis Society (USA) Advisory Committee on Clinical Trials of New Agents in Multiple Sclerosis. Neurology 1996;46:907-911.

18. Noseworthy JH, Lucchinetti C, Rodriguez M, Weinshenker BG. Multiple sclerosis. N Engl J Med 2000;343:938-952.

19. Larochelle C, Uphaus T, Prat A, Zipp F. Secondary Progression in Multiple Sclerosis: Neuronal Exhaustion or Distinct Pathology? Trends Neurosci 2016;39:325-339.

20. Tutuncu M, Tang J, Zeid NA, et al. Onset of progressive phase is an age-dependent clinical milestone in multiple sclerosis. Multiple sclerosis 2013;19:188-198.

21. Lublin FD, Reingold SC, Cohen JA, et al. Defining the clinical course of multiple sclerosis: the 2013 revisions. Neurology 2014;83:278-286.

22. Lublin F. History of modern multiple sclerosis therapy. J Neurol 2005;252 Suppl 3:iii3-iii9.

23. Novartis. Extavia [online]. Available at: https://www.extavia.com/index.jsp?usertrack.filte r_applied=true&NovaId=2935377078060387042.

24. Biogen. Avonex [online]. Available at: https://www.avonex.com/?cid=ppc-ggl-gs-avone x-na-1-gs_avonex. Accessed 06/05/2017.

25. Biogen. Plegridy [online]. Available at: https://www.plegridy.com/. Accessed 06/05/ 2017.

26. EMDSerono. Rebif [online]. Available at: http://www.rebif.com/index?cmp=R_Branded+C ore_Core_Exact_Rebif_Google_PS&utm_source= google&utm_medium=cpc&utm_campaign=Bra nded%25252BCore&utm_content=Core_Exact& utm_term=Rebif&gclid=CjwKEAjwgtTJBRDRmd6 ZtLrGyxwSJAA7Fy-hgd2dM_1nHXdlmOtDlg7xu0 k-a9ECDaJrqhuklhseohoCbyTw_wcB. Accessed 06/05/2017.

27. Bayer. Betaseron [online]. Available at: https://www.betaseron.com/. Accessed 06/05/ 2017.

28. Paty DW, Li DK. Interferon beta-1b is effective in relapsing-remitting multiple sclerosis. II. MRI analysis results of a multicenter, randomized, double-blind, placebo-controlled trial. UBC MS/MRI Study Group and the IFNB Multiple Sclerosis Study Group. Neurology 1993;43:662-667.

29. Jacobs LD, Cookfair DL, Rudick RA, et al. A phase III trial of intramuscular recombinant interferon beta as treatment for exacerbating- remitting multiple sclerosis: design and conduct of study and baseline characteristics of patients. Multiple Sclerosis Collaborative Research Group (MSCRG). Mult Scler 1995;1:118-135.

30. Randomised double-blind placebo- controlled study of interferon beta-1a in relapsing/remitting multiple sclerosis. PRISMS (Prevention

of Relapses and Disability by Interferon beta-1a Subcutaneously in Multiple Sclerosis) Study Group. Lancet 1998;352:1498-1504.

31. Calabresi PA, Kieseier BC, Arnold DL, et al. Pegylated interferon beta-1a for relapsing- remitting multiple sclerosis (ADVANCE): a randomised, phase 3, double-blind study. Lancet Neurol 2014;13:657-665.

32. Teva. Copaxone [online]. Available at: https://www.copaxonehcp.com/. Accessed 06/ 05/2017.

33. Comi G, Cohen JA, Arnold DL, Wynn D, Filippi M, Group FS. Phase III dose-comparison study of glatiramer acetate for multiple sclerosis. Ann Neurol 2011;69:75-82.

34. Johnson KP, Brooks BR, Cohen JA, et al. Copolymer 1 reduces relapse rate and improves disability in relapsing-remitting multiple sclerosis: results of a phase III multicenter, double-blind placebo-controlled trial. The Copolymer 1 Multiple Sclerosis Study Group. Neurology 1995;45:1268-1276.

35. Biogen. Zinbryta [online]. Available at: https://www.zinbryta.com/?cid=ppc-ggl-branded-na-278-branded. Accessed 06/05/2017.

36. Kappos L, Wiendl H, Selmaj K, et al. Daclizumab HYP versus Interferon Beta-1a in Relapsing Multiple Sclerosis. N Engl J Med 2015;373:1418-1428.

37. Novartis. Gilenya [online]. Available at: http://www.gilenya.com/index.jsp. Accessed 06/ 05/2017.

38. Cohen JA, Barkhof F, Comi G, et al. Oral fingolimod or intramuscular interferon for relapsing multiple sclerosis. N Engl J Med 2010;362:402-415.

39. Sanofi-Genzyme. Aubagio [online]. Available at: https://www.aubagio.com/. Accessed 06/ 05/2017.

40. Miller AE, Wolinsky JS, Kappos L, et al. Oral teriflunomide for patients

with a first clinical episode suggestive of multiple sclerosis (TOPIC): a randomised, double-blind, placebo-controlled, phase 3 trial. Lancet Neurol 2014;13:977-986.

41. O'Connor P, Wolinsky JS, Confavreux C, et al. Randomized trial of oral teriflunomide for relapsing multiple sclerosis. N Engl J Med 2011;365:1293-1303.

42. Confavreux C, O'Connor P, Comi G, et al. Oral teriflunomide for patients with relapsing multiple sclerosis (TOWER): a randomised, double- blind, placebo-controlled, phase 3 trial. Lancet Neurol 2014;13:247-256.

43. Biogen. Tecfidera [online]. Available at: https://www.tecfidera.com/. Accessed 06/05/ 2017.

44. Fox R, Miller DH, Phillips JT, et al. Placebo- controlled phase 3 study of oral BG-12 or glatiramer in multiple sclerosis. N Engl J Med 2012;367(12):1087-97.

45. Singh SK, Ruzek D. Neuroviral infections. General principles and DNA viruses. Boca Raton: CRC Press/Taylor & Francis, 2013.

46. Cettomai D, Pulicken M, Gordon-Lipkin E, et al. Reproducibility of optical coherence tomography in multiple sclerosis. Archives of neurology 2008;65:1218-1222.

47. Polman CH, O'Connor PW, Havrdova E, et al. A randomized, placebo-controlled trial of natalizumab for relapsing multiple sclerosis. N Engl J Med 2006;354:899-910.

48. Sanofi-Genzyme. Lemtrada [online]. Available at: https://www.lemtradahcp.com/. Accessed 06/05/2017.

49. Cohen JA, Coles AJ, Arnold DL, et al. Alemtuzumab versus interferon beta 1a as first-line treatment for patients with relapsing-remitting multiple sclerosis: a randomised controlled phase 3 trial. Lancet 2012;380:1819-1828.

50. Coles AJ, Twyman CL, Arnold DL, et al. Alemtuzumab for patients with

relapsing multiple sclerosis after disease-modifying therapy: a randomised controlled phase 3 trial. Lancet 2012;380:1829-1839.

51. Giovannoni G, Cohen JA, Coles AJ, et al. Alemtuzumab improves preexisting disability in active relapsing-remitting MS patients. Neurology 2016;87:1985-1992.

52. Frohman EM, Fujimoto JG, Frohman TC, Calabresi PA, Cutter G, Balcer LJ. Optical coherence tomography: a window into the mechanisms of multiple sclerosis. Nature clinical practice Neurology 2008;4:664-675.

53. Hauser SL, Bar-Or A, Comi G, et al. Ocrelizumab versus Interferon Beta-1a in Relapsing Multiple Sclerosis. N Engl J Med 2017;376:221-234.

54. Montalban X, Hauser SL, Kappos L, et al. Ocrelizumab versus Placebo in Primary Progressive Multiple Sclerosis. The New England journal of medicine 2017;376:209-220.

55. Young IR, Hall AS, Pallis CA, Legg NJ, Bydder GM, Steiner RE. Nuclear magnetic resonance imaging of the brain in multiple sclerosis. Lancet 1981;2:1063-1066.

56. Chen MYM, Pope TL, Ott DJ. Basic radiology : a Lange medical book. New York: Lange Medical Books/McGraw-Hill, Medical Pub. Div., 2004.

57. Grossman RI, Gonzalez-Scarano F, Atlas SW, Galetta S, Silberberg DH. Multiple sclerosis: gadolinium enhancement in MR imaging. Radiology 1986;161:721-725.

58. Gass A, Rocca MA, Agosta F, et al. MRI monitoring of pathological changes in the spinal cord in patients with multiple sclerosis. Lancet Neurol 2015;14:443-454.

59. Simon JH, Bermel RA, Rudick RA. Simple MRI metrics contribute to optimal care of the patient with multiple sclerosis. AJNR Am J Neuroradiol 2014;35:831-832.

60. Traboulsee A, Simon JH, Stone L, et al. Revised Recommendations of

the Consortium of MS Centers Task Force for a Standardized MRI Protocol and Clinical Guidelines for the Diagnosis and Follow-Up of Multiple Sclerosis. AJNR American journal of neuroradiology 2016;37:394-401.

61. Berkovich R. Treatment of acute relapses in multiple sclerosis. Neurotherapeutics 2013;10:97-105.

62. Lublin FD, Baier M, Cutter G. Effect of relapses on development of residual deficit in multiple sclerosis. Neurology 2003;61:1528-1532.

63. Filippini G, Brusaferri F, Sibley WA, et al. Corticosteroids or ACTH for acute exacerbations in multiple sclerosis. Cochrane Database Syst Rev 2000:CD001331.

64. Barnes D, Hughes RA, Morris RW, et al. Randomised trial of oral and intravenous methyl-prednisolone in acute relapses of multiple sclerosis. Lancet 1997;349:902-906.

65. Miller DM, Weinstock-Guttman B, Bethoux F, et al. A meta-analysis of methylprednisolone in recovery from multiple sclerosis exacerbations. Mult Scler 2000;6:267-273.

66. HealthUnionLLC. MS In America – relapse frequency and duration. [online]. Available at: https://multiplesclerosis.net/living-with-ms/multiple-sclerosis- relapses/ Accessed 06/06/2017.

67. Vollmer T. The natural history of relapses in multiple sclerosis. J Neurol Sci 2007;256 Suppl 1:S5-13.

68. Mallinckrodt. Acthar® Gel (Repository Corticotropin Injection) Prescribing Information. Mallinckrodt ARD Inc., 2015.

69. Kutz C. H.P. Acthar Gel (repository corticotropin injection) treatment of patients with multiple sclerosis and diabetes. Ther Adv Chronic Dis 2016;7:190-197.

70. Weinshenker BG. Therapeutic plasma exchange for acute inflammatory demyelinating syndromes of the central nervous system. J Clin Apher 1999;14:144-148.

71. Roed HG, Langkilde A, Sellebjerg F, et al. A double-blind, randomized trial of IV immuno-globulin treatment in acute optic neuritis. Neurology 2005;64:804-810.

72. Blight AR, Henney HR, 3rd, Cohen R. Development of dalfampridine, a novel pharmacologic approach for treating walking impairment in multiple sclerosis. Ann N Y Acad Sci 2014;1329:33-44.

73. Jeremy Ward RL. Physiology at a Glance: Wiley-Blackwell, 2013.

74. R.D Keynes DJA. Studies in Biology: Nerve and Muscle: Cambridge University Press.

75. Therapeutics A. Prescribing Information [online]. Available at: https://ampyra.com/prescribing-information.pdf. Accessed 06/07/2017.

76. Sharafaddinzadeh N, Moghtaderi A, Kashipazha D, Majdinasab N, Shalbafan B. The effect of low-dose naltrexone on quality of life of patients with multiple sclerosis: a randomized placebo-controlled trial. Mult Scler 2010;16:964-969.

77. Bowling AC. Complementary and alternative medicine in multiple sclerosis. Continuum (Minneap Minn) 2010;16:78-89.

78. Kevin Ergil ME. Fundamentals of Complementary and Alternative Medicine, Fifth Edition ed: Saunders, 2015.

79. Wang MY, Tsai PS, Lee PH, Chang WY, Yang CM. The efficacy of reflexology: systematic review. J Adv Nurs 2008;62:512-520.

80. Marijuana and the Cannabinoids: Humana Press, 2007.

81. Yadav V, Bever C, Jr., Bowen J, et al. Summary of evidence-based guideline: complementary and alternative medicine in multiple sclerosis: report of the guideline development subcommittee of the American Academy of Neurology. Neurology 2014;82:1083-1092.

82. Grigorian A, Araujo L, Naidu NN, Place DJ, Choudhury B, Demetriou

M. N- acetylglucosamine inhibits T-helper 1 (Th1)/T- helper 17 (Th17) cell responses and treats experimental autoimmune encephalomyelitis. J Biol Chem 2011;286:40133-40141.

83. Kanakasabai S, Casalini E, Walline CC, Mo C, Chearwae W, Bright JJ. Differential regulation of CD4(+) T helper cell responses by curcumin in experimental autoimmune encephalomyelitis. J Nutr Biochem 2012;23:1498-1507.

84. Sedel F, Papeix C, Bellanger A, et al. High doses of biotin in chronic progressive multiple sclerosis: a pilot study. Mult Scler Relat Disord 2015;4:159-169.

85. Tourbah A, Lebrun-Frenay C, Edan G, et al. MD1003 (high-dose biotin) for the treatment of progressive multiple sclerosis: A randomised, double-blind, placebo-controlled study. Multiple sclerosis 2016;22:1719-1731.

86. Evans E, Piccio L, Cross AH. Use of Vitamins and Dietary Supplements by Patients With Multiple Sclerosis: A Review. JAMA neurology 2018;75:1013-1021.

87. Hess MJ, Hess PE, Sullivan MR, Nee M, Yalla SV. Evaluation of cranberry tablets for the prevention of urinary tract infections in spinal cord injured patients with neurogenic bladder. Spinal Cord 2008;46:622-626.

88. Kranjcec B, Papes D, Altarac S. D- mannose powder for prophylaxis of recurrent urinary tract infections in women: a randomized clinical trial. World J Urol 2014;32:79-84.

89. Munger KL, Chitnis T, Ascherio A. Body size and risk of MS in two cohorts of US women. Neurology 2009;73:1543-1550.

90. O'Gorman C, Bukhari W, Todd A, Freeman S, Broadley SA. Smoking increases the risk of multiple sclerosis in Queensland, Australia. J Clin Neurosci 2014;21:1730-1733.

91. O'Gorman CM, Broadley SA. Smoking increases the risk of progression in multiple sclerosis: A cohort study in Queensland,

Australia. J Neurol Sci 2016;370:219-223.

92.   Riccio P, Rossano R. Nutrition facts in multiple sclerosis. ASN Neuro 2015;7.

93.   Muniz K. 20 ways Americans are blowing their money. USA Today 2014 March 24, 2014.

94.   Sardesai VM. Clinical Nutrition: CRC Press, 1998.

95.   Myles IA. Fast food fever: reviewing the impacts of the Western diet on immunity. Nutr J 2014;13:61.

96.   Thorburn AN, Macia L, Mackay CR. Diet, metabolites, and "western-lifestyle" inflammatory diseases. Immunity 2014;40:833-842.

97.   De Filippo C, Cavalieri D, Di Paola M, et al. Impact of diet in shaping gut microbiota revealed by a comparative study in children from Europe and rural Africa. Proc Natl Acad Sci U S A 2010;107:14691-14696.

98.   Bellik Y, Boukraa L, Alzahrani HA, et al. Molecular mechanism underlying anti-inflammatory and anti-allergic activities of phytochemicals: an update. Molecules 2012;18:322-353.

99.   Hever J. Plant-Based Diets: A Physician's Guide. Perm J 2016;20:93-101.

100.   Shor DB, Barzilai O, Ram M, et al. Gluten sensitivity in multiple sclerosis: experimental myth or clinical truth? Ann N Y Acad Sci 2009;1173:343-349.

101.   Reichelt KL, Jensen D. IgA antibodies against gliadin and gluten in multiple sclerosis. Acta Neurol Scand 2004;110:239-241.

102.   Stefferl A, Schubart A, Storch M, et al. Butyrophilin, a milk protein, modulates the encephalitogenic T cell response to myelin oligodendrocyte glycoprotein in experimental autoimmune encephalomyelitis. J Immunol 2000;165:2859-2865.

103. Kleinewietfeld M, Manzel A, Titze J, et al. Sodium chloride drives autoimmune disease by the induction of pathogenic TH17 cells. Nature 2013;496:518-522.

104. Wu C, Yosef N, Thalhamer T, et al. Induction of pathogenic TH17 cells by inducible salt-sensing kinase SGK1. Nature 2013;496:513-517.

105. Zostawa J, Adamczyk J, Sowa P, Adamczyk-Sowa M. The influence of sodium on pathophysiology of multiple sclerosis. Neurol Sci 2017;38:389-398.

106. Fitzgerald KC, Munger KL, Hartung HP, et al. Sodium intake and multiple sclerosis activity and progression in BENEFIT. Ann Neurol 2017.

107. Van Horn L, Carson JA, Appel LJ, et al. Recommended Dietary Pattern to Achieve Adherence to the American Heart Association/ American College of Cardiology (AHA/ACC) Guidelines: A Scientific Statement From the American Heart Association. Circulation 2016;134:e505-e529.

108. Finamore A, Palmery M, Bensehaila S, Peluso I. Antioxidant, Immunomodulating, and Microbial-Modulating Activities of the Sustainable and Ecofriendly Spirulina. Oxid Med Cell Longev 2017;2017:3247528.

109. Hudson JB. Applications of the phytomedicine Echinacea purpurea (Purple Coneflower) in infectious diseases. J Biomed Biotechnol 2012;2012:769896.

110. Li M, Yan YX, Yu QT, et al. Comparison of Immunomodulatory Effects of Fresh Garlic and Black Garlic Polysaccharides on RAW 264.7 Macrophages. J Food Sci 2017;82:765-771.

111. Neish AS. Microbes in gastrointestinal health and disease. Gastroenterology 2009;136:65-80.

112. Wu GD, Chen J, Hoffmann C, et al. Linking long-term dietary patterns with gut microbial enterotypes. Science 2011;334:105-108.

113. Berer K, Mues M, Koutrolos M, et al. Commensal microbiota and myelin autoantigen cooperate to trigger autoimmune demyelination. Nature 2011;479:538-541.

114. Jorg S, Grohme DA, Erzler M, et al. Environmental factors in autoimmune diseases and their role in multiple sclerosis. Cell Mol Life Sci 2016;73:4611-4622.

115. Galley JD, Bailey MT. Impact of stressor exposure on the interplay between commensal microbiota and host inflammation. Gut Microbes 2014;5:390-396.

116. Chassaing B, Gewirtz AT. Gut microbiota, low-grade inflammation, and metabolic syndrome. Toxicol Pathol 2014;42:49-53.

117. Issazadeh-Navikas S, Teimer R, Bockermann R. Influence of dietary components on regulatory T cells. Mol Med 2012;18:95-110.

118. Kosiewicz MM, Zirnheld AL, Alard P. Gut microbiota, immunity, and disease: a complex relltionship. Front Microbiol 2011;2:180.

119. Thomas F, Hehemann JH, Rebuffet E, Czjzek M, Michel G. Environmental and gut bacteroidetes: the food connection. Front Microbiol 2011;2:93.

120. Desvergne B, Michalik L, Wahli W. Transcriptional regulation of metabolism. Physiol Rev 2006;86:465-514.

121. Swank RL. Multiple sclerosis; a correlation of its incidence with dietary fat. Am J Med Sci 1950;220:421-430.

122. Swank RL, Goodwin J. Review of MS patient survival on a Swank low saturated fat diet. Nutrition 2003;19:161-162.

123. Maffei M, Halaas J, Ravussin E, et al. Leptin levels in human and rodent: measurement of plasma leptin and ob RNA in obese and weight- reduced subjects. Nat Med 1995;1:1155-1161.

124. Mohamed-Ali V, Goodrick S, Rawesh A, et al. Subcutaneous adipose

tissue releases interleukin-6, but not tumor necrosis factor-alpha, in vivo. J Clin Endocrinol Metab 1997;82:4196-4200.

125. Wang S, Moustaid-Moussa N, Chen L, et al. Novel insights of dietary polyphenols and obesity. J Nutr Biochem 2014;25:1-18.

126. Gupta SC, Tyagi AK, Deshmukh-Taskar P, Hinojosa M, Prasad S, Aggarwal BB. Downregulation of tumor necrosis factor and other proinflammatory biomarkers by polyphenols. Arch Bio-chem Biophys 2014;559:91-99.

127. Scalbert A, Manach C, Morand C, Remesy C, Jimenez L. Dietary polyphenols and the prevention of diseases. Crit Rev Food Sci Nutr 2005;45:287-306.

128. Wright N, Wilson L, Smith M, Duncan B, McHugh P. The BROAD study: A randomised controlled trial using a whole food plant-based diet in the community for obesity, ischaemic heart disease or diabetes. Nutr Diabetes 2017;7:e256.

129. Esselstyn CB, Jr., Gendy G, Doyle J, Golubic M, Roizen MF. A way to reverse CAD? J Fam Pract 2014;63:356-364b.

130. Turner-McGrievy GM, Barnard ND, Scialli AR. A two-year randomized weight loss trial comparing a vegan diet to a more moderate low-fat diet. Obesity (Silver Spring) 2007;15:2276-2281.

131. Promotion TOoDPaH. Dietary Guidelines for Americans 2015-20202015.

132. Pedersen BK, Saltin B. Evidence for prescribing exercise as therapy in chronic disease. Scand J Med Sci Sports 2006;16 Suppl 1:3-63.

133. Mostert S, Kesselring J. Effects of a short- term exercise training program on aerobic fitness, fatigue, health perception and activity level of subjects with multiple sclerosis. Mult Scler 2002;8:161-168.

134. Dalgas U, Stenager E, Ingemann-Hansen T. Multiple sclerosis and physical exercise: recommendations for the application of resistance, endurance and combined training. Mult Scler

2008;14:35-53.

135. Sabapathy NM, Minahan CL, Turner GT, Broadley SA. Comparing endurance andand resistance exercise training in people with multiple sclerosis: a randomized pilot study. Clin Rehabil 2011;25:14-24.

136. Layne JE, Nelson ME. The effects of progressive resistance training on bone density: a review. Med Sci Sports Exerc 1999;31:25-30.

137. Speakman JR, Selman C. Physical activity and resting metabolic rate. Proc Nutr Soc 2003;62:621-634.

138. Elan D. Louis SAM, Lewis P. Rowland. Merritt's Neurology. Philadelphia, PA: Wolters Kluwer, 2016.

139. Campbell WW. DeJong's The Neurological Examination. Philadelphia, PA: Wolters Kluwer, 2013.

140. Herring MP, Fleming KM, Hayes SP, Motl RW, Coote SB. Moderators of Exercise Effects on Depressive Symptoms in Multiple Sclerosis: A Meta-regression. Am J Prev Med 2017.

141. McHugh MP, Cosgrave CH. To stretch or not to stretch: the role of stretching in injury prevention and performance. Scand J Med Sci Sports 2010;20:169-181.

142. The Health Consequences of Smoking-50 Years of Progress: A Report of the Surgeon General. Atlanta (GA)2014.

143. Correale J, Farez MF. Smoking worsens multiple sclerosis prognosis: two different pathways are involved. J Neuroimmunol 2015;281:23-34.

144. Wingerchuk DM. Smoking: effects on multiple sclerosis susceptibility and disease progression. Ther Adv Neurol Disord 2012;5:13-22.

145. Van Schayck OCP, Williams S, Barchilon V, et al. Treating tobacco dependence: guidance for primary care on life-saving

interventions. Position statement of the IPCRG. NPJ Prim Care Respir Med 2017;27:38.

146. Patnode CD, Henderson JT, Thompson JH, Senger CA, Fortmann SP, Whitlock EP. Behavioral Counseling and Pharmacotherapy Interventions for Tobacco Cessation in Adults, Including Pregnant Women: A Review of Reviews for the U.S. Preventive Services Task Force. Ann Intern Med 2015;163:608-621.

147. Goyal M, Singh S, Sibinga EM, et al. Meditation programs for psychological stress and well- being: a systematic review and meta-analysis. JAMA Intern Med 2014;174:357-368.

148. Fisk JD, Pontefract A, Ritvo PG, Archibald CJ, Murray TJ. The impact of fatigue on patients with multiple sclerosis. Can J Neurol Sci 1994;21:9-14.

149. Vucic S, Burke D, Kiernan MC. Fatigue in multiple sclerosis: mechanisms and management. Clin Neurophysiol 2010;121:809-817.

150. Kos D, Kerckhofs E, Nagels G, D'Hooghe M B, Ilsbroukx S. Origin of fatigue in multiple sclerosis: review of the literature. Neurorehabil Neural Repair 2008;22:91-100.

151. Langeskov-Christensen M, Bisson EJ, Finlayson ML, Dalgas U. Potential pathophysiological pathways that can explain the positive effects of exercise on fatigue in multiple sclerosis: A scoping review. J Neurol Sci 2017;373:307-320.

152. Krupp LB, Coyle PK, Doscher C, et al. Fatigue therapy in multiple sclerosis: results of a double-blind, randomized, parallel trial of amantadine, pemoline, and placebo. Neurology 1995;45:1956-1961.

153. Zifko UA. Management of fatigue in patients with multiple sclerosis. Drugs 2004;64:1295-1304.

154. Bamer AM, Johnson KL, Amtmann D, Kraft GH. Prevalence of sleep problems in individuals with multiple sclerosis. Mult Scler

2008;14:1127-1130.

155. Boe Lunde HM, Aae TF, Indrevag W, et al. Poor sleep in patients with multiple sclerosis. PLoS One 2012;7:e49996.

156. Brass SD, Li CS, Auerbach S. The underdiagnosis of sleep disorders in patients with multiple sclerosis. J Clin Sleep Med 2014;10:1025-1031.

157. Merlino G, Fratticci L, Lenchig C, et al. Prevalence of 'poor sleep' among patients with multiple sclerosis: an independent predictor of mental and physical status. Sleep Med 2009;10:26-34.

158. Carnicka Z, Kollar B, Siarnik P, Krizova L, Klobucnikova K, Turcani P. Sleep disorders in patients with multiple sclerosis. J Clin Sleep Med 2015;11:553-557.

159. Young T, Palta M, Dempsey J, Skatrud J, Weber S, Badr S. The occurrence of sleep- disordered breathing among middle-aged adults. N Engl J Med 1993;328:1230-1235.

160. Braley TJ, Segal BM, Chervin RD. Obstructive sleep apnea and fatigue in patients with multiple sclerosis. J Clin Sleep Med 2014;10:155-162.

161. Aburub A, Khalil H, Al-Sharman A, Alomari M, Khabour O. The association between physical activity and sleep characteristics in people with multiple sclerosis. Mult Scler Relat Disord 2017;12:29-33.

162. Caffeine for the Sustainment of Mental Task Performance: Formulations for Military Operations. Washington (DC)2001.

163. Drulovic J, Basic-Kes V, Grgic S, et al. The Prevalence of Pain in Adults with Multiple Sclerosis: A Multicenter Cross-Sectional Survey. Pain Med 2015;16:1597-1602.

164. O'Connor AB, Schwid SR, Herrmann DN, Markman JD, Dworkin RH. Pain associated with multiple sclerosis: systematic review and proposed classification. Pain 2008;137:96-111.

165. Tuzun E, Akman-Demir G, Eraksoy M. Paroxysmal attacks in multiple sclerosis. Mult Scler 2001;7:402-404.

166. Al-Araji AH, Oger J. Reappraisal of Lhermitte's sign in multiple sclerosis. Mult Scler 2005;11:398-402.

167. Cruccu G. Trigeminal Neuralgia. Continuum (Minneap Minn) 2017;23:396-420.

168. Pollmann W, Feneberg W. Current management of pain associated with multiple sclerosis. CNS Drugs 2008;22:291-324.

169. Flachenecker P, Henze T, Zettl UK. Spasticity in patients with multiple sclerosis clinical characteristics, treatment and quality of life. Acta Neurol Scand 2014;129:154-162.

170. Cheung J, Rancourt A, Di Poce S, et al. Patient-identified factors that influence spasticity in people with stroke and multiple sclerosis receiving botulinum toxin injection treatments. Physiother Can 2015;67:157-166.

171. Backus D, Manella C, Bender A, Sweatman M. Impact of Massage Therapy on Fatigue, Pain, and Spasticity in People with Multiple Sclerosis: a Pilot Study. Int J Ther Massage Bodywork 2016;9:4-13.

172. Hyman N, Barnes M, Bhakta B, et al. Botulinum toxin (Dysport) treatment of hip adductor spasticity in multiple sclerosis: a prospective, randomised, double blind, placebo controlled, dose ranging study. J Neurol Neurosurg Psychiatry 2000;68:707-712.

173. Otero-Romero S, Sastre-Garriga J, Comi G, et al. Pharmacological management of spasticity in multiple sclerosis: Systematic review and consensus paper. Mult Scler 2016;22:1386-1396.

174. Sandroff BM, Klaren RE, Motl RW. Relationships among physical inactivity, deconditioning, and walking impairment in persons with multiple sclerosis. J Neurol Phys Ther 2015;39:103-110.

175. Chung LH, Remelius JG, Van Emmerik RE, Kent-Braun JA. Leg power

asymmetry and postural control in women with multiple sclerosis. Med Sci Sports Exerc 2008;40:1717-1724.

176. Sandroff BM, Sosnoff JJ, Motl RW. Physical fitness, walking performance, and gait in multiple sclerosis. J Neurol Sci 2013;328:70-76.

177. Chiaravalloti ND, DeLuca J. Cognitive impairment in multiple sclerosis. Lancet Neurol 2008;7:1139-1151.

178. Rao SM, Leo GJ, Bernardin L, Unverzagt F. Cognitive dysfunction in multiple sclerosis. I. Frequency, patterns, and prediction. Neurology 1991;41:685-691.

179. Rogers JM, Panegyres PK. Cognitive impairment in multiple sclerosis: evidence-based analysis and recommendations. J Clin Neurosci 2007;14:919-927.

180. Papathanasiou A, Messinis L, Georgiou VL, Papathanasopoulos P. Cognitive impairment in relapsing remitting and secondary progressive multiple sclerosis patients: efficacy of a computerized cognitive screening battery. ISRN Neurol 2014;2014:151379.

181. Papathanasiou A, Messinis L, Zampakis P, Papathanasopoulos P. Corpus callosum atrophy as a marker of clinically meaningful cognitive decline in secondary progressive multiple sclerosis. Impact on employment status. J Clin Neurosci 2017.

182. Lanz M, Hahn HK, Hildebrandt H. Brain atrophy and cognitive impairment in multiple sclerosis: a review. J Neurol 2007;254 Suppl 2:II43-48.

183. Benedict RH, Carone DA, Bakshi R. Correlating brain atrophy with cognitive dysfunction, mood disturbances, and personality disorder in multiple sclerosis. J Neuroimaging 2004;14:36S-45S.

184. Gustavsen MW, Celius EG, Winsvold BS, et al. Migraine and frequent tension-type headache are not associated with multiple sclerosis in a Norwegian case-control study. Mult Scler J Exp Transl Clin 2016;2:2055217316682976.

185. Putzki N, Pfriem A, Limmroth V, et al. Prevalence of migraine, tension-type headache and trigeminal neuralgia in multiple sclerosis. Eur J Neurol 2009;16:262-267.

186. Pollmann W, Erasmus LP, Feneberg W, Then Bergh F, Straube A. Interferon beta but not glatiramer acetate therapy aggravates headaches in MS. Neurology 2002;59:636-639.

187. Goldman Consensus G. The Goldman Consensus statement on depression in multiple sclerosis. Mult Scler 2005;11:328-337.

188. Feinstein A. Multiple sclerosis and depression. Mult Scler 2011;17:1276-1281.

189. Minden SL, Feinstein A, Kalb RC, et al. Evidence-based guideline: assessment and management of psychiatric disorders in individuals with MS: report of the Guideline Development Subcommittee of the American Academy of Neurology. Neurology 2014;82:174-181.

190. Fishman I, Benedict RH, Bakshi R, Priore R, Weinstock-Guttman B. Construct validity and frequency of euphoria sclerotica in multiple sclerosis. J Neuropsychiatry Clin Neurosci 2004;16:350-356.

191. Hammond FM, Alexander DN, Cutler AJ, et al. PRISM II: an open-label study to assess effectiveness of dextromethorphan/quinidine for pseudobulbar affect in patients with dementia, stroke or traumatic brain injury. BMC Neurol 2016;16:89.

192. Ahmed A, Simmons Z. Pseudobulbar affect: prevalence and management. Ther Clin Risk Manag 2013;9:483-489.

193. Pioro EP. Review of Dextromethorphan 20 mg/Quinidine 10 mg (NUEDEXTA((R))) for Pseudobulbar Affect. Neurol Ther 2014;3:15-28.

194. Adamec I, Habek M. Autonomic dysfunction in multiple sclerosis. Clin Neurol Neurosurg 2013;115 Suppl 1:S73-78.

195. Schurch B, Carda S. OnabotulinumtoxinA and multiple sclerosis. Ann Phys Rehabil Med 2014;57:302-314.

196. Wiesel PH, Norton C, Glickman S, Kamm MA. Pathophysiology and management of bowel dysfunction in multiple sclerosis. Eur J Gastroenterol Hepatol 2001;13:441-448.

197. Bronner G, Elran E, Golomb J, Korczyn AD. Female sexuality in multiple sclerosis: the multidimensional nature of the problem and the intervention. Acta Neurol Scand 2010;121:289-301.

198. Calabro RS, De Luca R, Conti-Nibali V, Reitano S, Leo A, Bramanti P. Sexual dysfunction in male patients with multiple sclerosis: a need for counseling! Int J Neurosci 2014;124:547-557.

199. Dehghan-Nayeri N, Khakbazan Z, Ghafoori F, Nabavi SM. Sexual dysfunction levels in iranian women suffering from multiple sclerosis. Mult Scler Relat Disord 2017;12:49-53.

200. Hulter BM, Lundberg PO. Sexual function in women with advanced multiple sclerosis. J Neurol Neurosurg Psychiatry 1995;59:83-86.

201. Baker DG. Multiple sclerosis and thermo- regulatory dysfunction. J Appl Physiol (1985) 2002;92:1779-1780.

202. Opara JA, Brola W, Wylegala AA, Wylegala E. Uhthoff`s phenomenon 125 years later - what do we know today? J Med Life 2016;9:101-105.

203. Vukusic S, Hutchinson M, Hours M, et al. Pregnancy and multiple sclerosis (the PRIMS study): clinical predictors of post-partum relapse. Brain : a journal of neurology 2004;127:1353-1360.

204. Roux T, Courtillot C, Debs R, Touraine P, Lubetzki C, Papeix C. Fecundity in women with multiple sclerosis: an observational mono-centric study. J Neurol 2015;262:957-960.

205. Coyle PK. Management of women with multiple sclerosis through pregnancy and after child- birth. Ther Adv Neurol Disord 2016;9:198-210.

206. Alroughani R, Altintas A, Al Jumah M, et al. Pregnancy and the Use of Disease-Modifying Therapies in Patients with Multiple Sclerosis: Benefits versus Risks. Mult Scler Int 2016;2016:1034912.

207. Almas S, Vance J, Baker T, Hale T. Management of Multiple Sclerosis in the Breastfeeding Mother. Mult Scler Int 2016;2016:6527458.

208. Brandt-Wouters E, Gerlach OH, Hupperts RM. The effect of postpartum intravenous immunoglobulins on the relapse rate among patients with multiple sclerosis. Int J Gynaecol Obstet 2016;134:194-196.

209. de Seze J, Chapelotte M, Delalande S, Ferriby D, Stojkovic T, Vermersch P. Intravenous corticosteroids in the postpartum period for reduction of acute exacerbations in multiple sclerosis. Mult Scler 2004;10:596-597.

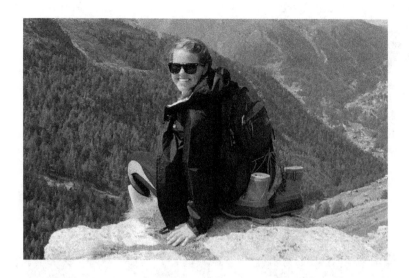

KATY WRIGHT, PA-C

Katy Wright, CPAS, PA-C, is a Physician Assistant in the Clinical Center for Multiple Sclerosis at the University of Texas Southwestern Medical Center in Dallas, Texas. Katy completed her undergraduate studies at Texas Tech University in Lubbock, Texas where she received her Bachelor of Science degree. She later earned her Master's of Physician Assistant Studies from the University of Texas Southwestern Medical Center School of Health Professionals in 2012. Katy is board certified as a Physician Assistant and has specialized in the treatment of MS since she entered the medical field.

In addition to her clinical responsibilities, Katy is involved in several research studies and clinical trials. She is a preceptor for visiting physician assistant and nurse practitioner students and a guest lecturer for the University of Texas Southwestern School of Health Professions' Physician Assistant Program.

Katy has a special interest in diet, exercise, and multidisciplinary care as she firmly believes that improving one's overall health optimizes their opportunities for success in managing their MS. She is currently pursuing a certification in holistic nutrition in an effort to better educate her patients on the importance of dietary choices and empower them to make positive health behavior changes. She is the author of a mobile application that serves as a transition guide and recipe database for those pursuing a whole food, plant- based diet. Katy is also the Executive Producer of the documentary *Multiple Seasons*, an effort aimed at redefining MS and demonstrating how a single individual with an orphan disease like MS can be the catalyst for positive change for an entire community.

Katy is a Fellow of the American Academy of Physician Assistants, Fellow of the Texas Academy of Physician Assistants, and a member of the American Academy of Neurology.

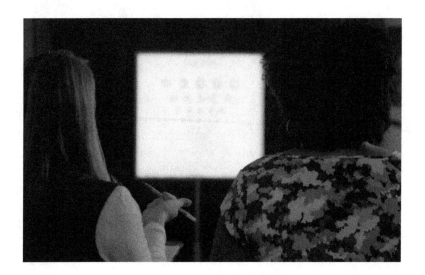

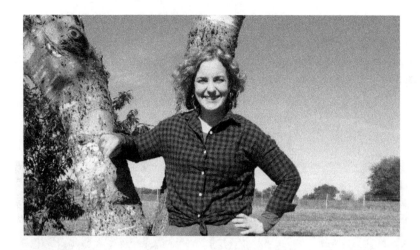

MANDY WINKLER, RN

Mandy Winkler, RN, BSN, is a Registered Nurse at the University of Texas Southwestern Medical Center Clinical Center for Multiple Sclerosis Clinic in Dallas, Texas. Mandy received her Bachelor of Science degree from Oklahoma Baptist University in Shawnee, Oklahoma. Following graduation, she worked in the cardiac ICU before transitioning to an outpatient ENT clinic. She has worked in the field of multiple sclerosis for the past 5 years. Mandy is passionate about educating patients and their care partners about MS. She has a special interest in health and wellness and currently serves as the fitness coordinator for the upcoming documentary *Multiple Seasons*. She was a collaborator for Bring Healthcare Back Home; a community service initiative funded by the MS Foundation that allowed patients to receive multidisciplinary care in their home.

She is a member of the International Organization of Multiple Sclerosis Nurses and American Academy of Neurology. Mandy was a finalist for the Dallas Magazine Excellence in Nursing award in 2015 and received the Diana and Richard C. Strauss Service Excellence Award in 2017.

In addition to her clinical responsibilities, she is involved in 3 different clinical trials and investigator initiated research. She also serves as the primary investigator for her own study, examining the underserved patient populations within Hawaii. Mandy has a strong desire to pursue excellence and continually strives to increase her breadth of knowledge in an effort to better serve her patients.

Mandy has also served as a leader in her local church and been actively involved in both domestic and international mission work. God is her source of strength, joy, and is the driving force behind her passion to help others.

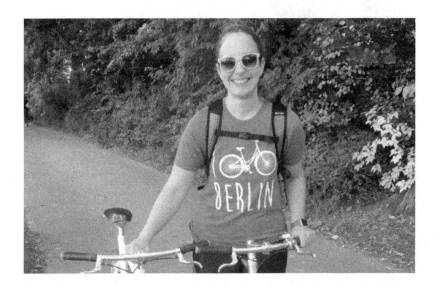

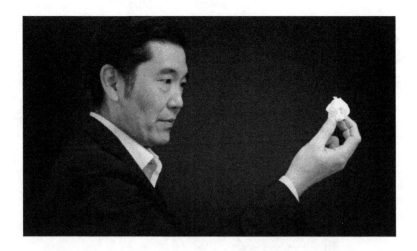

DARIN T. OKUDA, MD, MS, FAAN, FANA

Dr. Okuda is a clinician-scientist and professor specializing in multiple sclerosis within the Department of Neurology and Neurotherapeutics at UT Southwestern Medical Center in Dallas, Texas. Dr. Okuda completed his undergraduate, graduate, and medical education at the University of Hawaii. Following his residency training in neurology he completed a fellowship in neuroimmunology at the University of California, San Francisco Multiple Sclerosis Center. Within UT Southwestern, he currently serves as Director of the Neuroinnovation Program, Director of the Multiple Sclerosis and Neuroimmunology Imaging Program, and Deputy Director of the MS Program at the Clinical Center for Multiple Sclerosis.

Dr. Okuda's current focus involves end-to-end innovative approaches involving the design, creation and implementation of tools aimed at improving the evaluation, diagnosis, and management of patients with multiple sclerosis and other neurological diseases. He is both nationally and internationally recognized for his work in defining and investigating radiologically isolated syndrome (RIS) and currently directs scientific strategies within the Radiologically Isolated Syndrome Consortium (RISC), a multi-national working group aimed at advancing the science within the very early forms of CNS demyelination. His work is also focused on creating next generation healthcare by designing innovative connections between patients and providers, developing new diagnostic and clinical surveillance metrics, transforming medical decision-making, and challenging existing norms. He continues to be actively involved in extreme healthcare efforts aimed at delivering care more accurately, efficiently, and intelligently.

Dr. Okuda is a Diplomate of The American Board of Psychiatry and Neurology, Inc., Fellow of the American Academy of Neurology, Fellow of the American Neurological Association, and member of the American Academy of Neurology Committees on Neuro-imaging and Ethics.

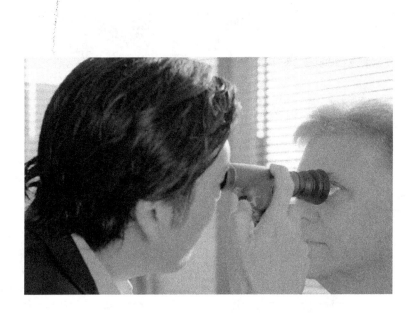

CPSIA information can be obtained
at www.ICGtesting.com
Printed in the USA
BVHW011334080319
542173BV00010B/74/P